MW00366054

FIELD GUIDE TO TEACHING YOGA

Overcoming Fears, Rising to Challenges, and Thriving in a Job You Love

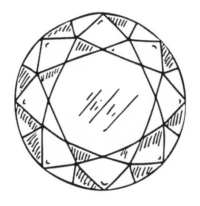

By: Jackie Kinealy

Printed in the United States of America.

Cover Design by Blaise Hart-Schmidt.

First edition, 2019.

ISBN: 9781082891038

www.jakyoga.com

CONTENTS

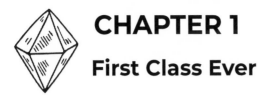

CHAPTER 1

First Class Ever

"The expert at anything
was once a beginner."

-Helen Hayes

Five minutes before teaching my first yoga class, I was trying to look natural and professional by reorganizing the props in the studio that I had rented for the hour. No one had shown up for the class yet, and as I refolded a stack of Mexican blankets, I prayed nobody would.

Earlier in the day, I was nervous but optimistic. I had just moved to town, and I didn't know anybody except my then-boyfriend, now-husband, Dan. He was supposed to come to class as moral support but had texted 30 minutes earlier to say he was really sorry, but he was stuck at a city council meeting, and I would do great.

Deep breath. *That's okay*, I thought. I had spent the three weeks leading up to this night tacking fliers and free class cards on coffee shop boards and lamp posts. Of all the people who saw them, I figured at least five or six would come.

Right?

Wrong, it seemed. The class was supposed to start at 7 pm. Now it was 6:57 and I was alone. I had switched from stacking the blankets to sorting some papers at the front desk that were not mine. Meanwhile, new-age flute music played softly in the background.

At least if nobody showed up I could be embarrassed and disappointed in private—switch my Spotify to Fleetwood Mac and dance out my feelings. It would be cathartic! But if one person came, I would have to teach a terribly awkward class to a stranger, my armpits itchy with stage-fright, trying to pretend I felt confident and calm when in reality I was certain that she could tell I had no idea what I was doing, that I had no business teaching yoga.

Then at 6:58 pm, a woman carrying a yoga mat walked in. Instantly, my armpits prickled and my face got hot. She frowned into the empty studio and asked, "Is there yoga class tonight?"

I tried to smile with confidence, "Yep, you're in the right place!" I said. "We'll get started in a couple of minutes! Just get comfortable!!" I escorted her to the shelf of props—impeccably stacked—while inside I died a little.

Walking back to the front desk, I gave myself a pep talk, tried to adjust to the fact that someone was actually freaking here to take a yoga class that I was teaching. *This is fine, you're fine! This will be great! It's cool! She doesn't think you're a loser!* I opened my notebook and stared at my class plan. *Why wasn't I doing this before instead of messing up someone else's papers?!* Meanwhile, the lone student unrolled her mat in the center of the huge studio, and sat on the floor, looking a bit uneasy.

Then, praise Jesus, a second woman walked in the door just as the clock clicked to 7 pm. I felt a drop in my chest that was similar to a feeling of relief, except there was no decrease in anxiety along with it. Two students wasn't a great class, but it was better than one! Same as before, I showed her to the props and the yoga room. Then, for some reason, I did a little bow. It was weird. At 7:01, it was time to start. I grabbed my class plan notebook and followed her inside.

How I Got Here

Eight years earlier, at the first yoga class I took at my college gym, I instantly loved it. I tingled with peacefulness after class. I had never experienced anything quite like the feeling, but it was similar to one night in third grade when my mom slowly traced the outline of my body on a long strip of butcher paper and I could feel all my edges at once, and also a day in high school when our religion teacher taught us Tai Chi on the first warm day of spring and I could feel a ball of energy between my palms. Right away, I knew I had discovered something special in yoga, something brand new and deeply familiar at the same time.

Still, my practice didn't take root for a few years. I practiced at home only a handful of times and attended classes sporadically. That changed when I moved to Colorado after college. Seeking a community there and something to do after work, I discovered a yoga studio that offered a free class on Thursday nights, taught by a man named Kirk who was so passionate and dorky and awesome. Every class had an inspirational theme, which he would describe with vigor, almost like a preacher. "The dragonfly! Is the most...ancient...insect!" he began one dark winter evening, "They symbolize. Transformation. *You* are dragonflies."

Yes, I was! I loved that class; I rarely missed a week. It was a place I could go between my job in a cavernous, overly air-conditioned office and the 600-square-foot, unairconditioned apartment that I shared with my best friend. Yoga made my body feel strong and good and healthy. I was calm and happy. My life felt spiritual and significant. Like magic, I figured out things about my life during class; answers to my questions would come clear.

I wanted more of that. I wanted to teach. I wanted to do what Kirk did—create a yoga church for people in the hour between work and dinner. I'm supposed to say that I wanted to become a yoga teacher in order to help people and make a positive contribution to the world, but I don't think that is quite true. Nowadays, it is true, but it wasn't the main reason at the time. I wanted to become a yoga teacher for *me*, because I *loved* it with a burning flame, because I felt a calling, and because I had a feeling that I could be good at it. Whenever I left a class, I would sit in the parking lot scribbling in my notebook ideas for class themes, metaphors about tree pose (which I'm sure were super insightful), imagery that would be good to use in *savasana*. Eight years after my first class, and two years after I had embarked on a near-obsessive yoga practice, I signed up for a month-long 200-hour training.

The program was not, how do you say...good. The facilitator was goodhearted and sweet, but not an effective trainer. She was spacey and disorganized. She arrived 15 minutes late on the first day of the training; the group of us were locked outside the studio wondering what was up. Another day we caravanned to a cafe where we spent a whole morning eating pastries, which were tasty, but not what I signed up for. Sometimes when one of us asked a question, you could see her panic at not knowing the answer and abruptly change the subject. After that happened a few times, some people in the group started to press her for an answer, acting more like reporters than yoga students, "You didn't answer the question!" By the end of the second week, things had deteriorated to a point that I worried there might be a mutiny.

There was not a mutiny, but it was still pretty bad. We simply weren't learning enough. Each of us led only two practice classes, a short one and a long one, and we devoted very little time to anatomy and modifications. The portion about yoga philosophy was cursory. We just memorized, and quickly forgot, the *yamas* and the *niyamas*. It is probably not surprising that the program is now defunct. In fact, there was a scary moment when I was applying for my 300-hour training when my application got flagged because the admissions people couldn't find my 200-hour training in the Yoga Alliance directory.

Back to My First Class Ever

All this to say that during that first class I was equal parts burning ball of passion—because I was starting to live my dream—and bone-deep anxiety because I had zero confidence in my authority as a yoga teacher. Quite the combo. That first night, I don't remember my sequence or theme, but I do remember feeling so nervous that I didn't smile or make eye contact the entire time, not even at the beginning or end of class, which must have been strange for them. I was so focused on teaching exactly what I had written in my notebook that I barely noticed if they were following along. It was like we weren't in the same room.

It was not pretty, but then finally it was over. The two women left, and I was again alone in the studio, feeling the dazed relief of someone who just drove through a blizzard for an hour. I biked home, poured a glass of wine, and waited for Dan to get back from that dumb city council meeting. The next week, I did the whole thing again: the props and papers, the ambient music, the sweaty pits, the weird lack of eye contact, the glass of wine. Week after week, I woke up with low-grade anxiety that didn't resolve until class wrapped up that night.

Despite it all, I still really loved teaching yoga, and I felt like I was on the right path. The more I taught, the more I realized just how much I didn't know. I started studying, reading, and taking online courses like crazy. I also started teaching two more classes—one at a community center for disabled adults and the other in the attic of a historic building downtown (Calvin Coolidge once had his law office there!). As for the community center class, it was a joy. It was silly, fun, low-pressure and a great way to learn how to modify for different people. The attic class was good because I didn't have to pay for it. Instead, I would mop and clean after class each week in exchange for the hour. Students paid by donation, and some weeks I would actually walk away with $70 or $80. I am still grateful to the retired couple who gave me $40 every week. Because I still had a day job, pubescent money-management skills, and a subconscious belief that I didn't really deserve to be paid for teaching yoga, the money I earned felt like a fun bonus, and Dan and I would often spend it at restaurants immediately after class.

Things improved a little, but honestly, my first year was mostly a hot mess. I did gradually feel more comfortable teaching—the fact that the same people came back each week gave me confidence—but still, I tingled with anxiety waiting for students to arrive. My actual teaching skills were stronger, but I interpreted any facial expression that hinted something other than complete and total absorption as a sign that I was doing a horrible job. Eventually, I could look around the room at people, but when I did I often saw students who were clearly uncomfortable in Downward Dog—backs rounded, weight dumping forward, heads lifting—but I was stumped. I couldn't figure out what specifically to tell them that would help. Even though I was doing hours of studying and reading each week, I tensed when students asked me questions after class, nervous that I wouldn't know the answer would be exposed as a fraud.

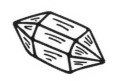

You Are Not Alone

Bottom line: I didn't know what I was doing, and I felt alone because I didn't realize that it's *normal* to feel that way when you start a new job. Of *course* it is! Imagine talking with a friend at the end of her first week working as an ICU nurse, and she says she feels totally overwhelmed and unqualified to care for actual patients, instead of just learning about it in nursing school. Unless you are a mean friend, you would probably reassure her that it's completely normal and she will feel much better in six months.

Teaching yoga is no different. Sure, it's less intense than the ICU, but you should still give yourself the same permission to ride the learning curve that you would give a friend starting a new job as a nurse, high school teacher, accountant, or weatherman.

In some ways, being a new yoga teacher is harder than those jobs because usually after your teacher training program you are on your own. You have to figure out how to make a job of it with little to no mentorship, guidance, or formal feedback. The ICU nurse, at least, is surrounded by other nurses and doctors who can answer her questions. For accountants, there are internships, where you get experience in a real office. When a rookie weatherman messes up with the green screen, it's adorable and someone puts it on a blooper compilation on YouTube.

Meanwhile, the profession of teaching yoga seriously lacks a meaningful support structure for people after they teacher training. Certainly, there are exceptions: some studios provide a set sequence for new teachers while they develop their teaching muscles. But elsewhere, it's all or nothing. You finish training, and the next step is to start teaching classes, which feels more like a giant leap than a step. You can't get an entry level job or an internship to get your feet wet; you have to grab onto the rope swing, get a running start, and jump into the lake.

You Can Do It!

I wrote this book to help fill the gap between finishing your YTT program and feeling ready to actually teach. This book distills what I have learned from going through the experience myself, feeling totally unprepared to teach classes and doing it anyway. I wrote what I have learned from teaching a couple of thousand hours of yoga classes in the past five years. I am close enough to the experience to remember it honestly, and far enough away to assure you that it gets so much better.

First, I hope this book fortifies you with the knowledge that you are not alone in feeling freaked out, shy, unsure, and scared. It's normal. You are normal (well, at least when it come to this), and you are great. You won't always feel overwhelmed, but you probably will for at least a year. Keep teaching, keep working hard, and you will get through it.

Second, I hope this book helps you do your best work: to sharpen your skills, stay in a healthy mindset, plan your future career, develop a plan to grow your classes, and help students get the most out of their practice.

Last, and most of all, I hope that this book helps you actually teach yoga to people. I hope it helps you get through the intimidation, the fear, and the not knowing where to start. I hope it connects you with your love of yoga, which inspired you to teach in the first place. I hope this book can carry you over the choppy waters of your first year, to a patch of solid ground on the other side: a bridge between your teacher training and your best teaching.

I started this book project as a brand-new teacher who felt anxious and unsure in the classroom, who spent hours each week planning three classes, who was scared that her students hated her, and who occasionally taught some messy classes. At the same time, I am sure I also taught plenty of classes that I thought were terrible, but were actually fine. Five years later, I am finishing this project as a yoga teacher who feels confident and comfortable most of the time. I worry less about every student liking me, and I don't take it personally if a lady has resting-bitch-face during class, or is staring at the ceiling in *savasana*.

One of the biggest improvements is that I am present in the room with my students, instead of inside my own head. I smile now! I look people in the eye! But not constantly! That's also weird! I am comfortable enough to notice how people are actually doing, walk around the room, and offer help.

I have my dream job, teaching full-time at a studio where I love my students and coworkers. I get to create and lead workshops, retreats, and teacher training. Yes, I still have so much to learn, but that's exciting, and I have time and support to study, practice, and develop as an instructor.

Most importantly, I feel a deep sense of pleasure and purpose in my work. Back in Colorado when I first felt that teaching yoga was my calling. I do believe I was right. Teaching yoga is the work I'm meant to do. If you're reading this book, you're probably saying, "Yes! Me too!" and if you're saying that, you should keep going. Don't abandon your calling. I love what I do. I believe it makes a real difference for people; yoga can change the world, truly. Also, it is simply a great job, one that is fun and refreshing and creative and spiritual and friendly and satisfying and awesome.

Let me tell you one more thing about that first class. Those two women who were on board for that bumpy ride? They came back. Most weeks, actually. They ended up being my two most consistent students. The lesson is not that I was actually amazing from the start, but I just couldn't see it. Rather, the lesson is that I didn't need to take myself so seriously. They either didn't notice how much I was struggling, or they didn't care. In general, people are thinking way more about their own experience than yours. In yoga class, folks just want to move, and stretch, and breathe, and get quiet and still. Give them the chance to do that, and your class will be fine.

Let's get started.

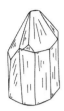

CHAPTER 2

Three Essential Mindsets

"Calm yourself, believe in yourself,
stick to your routine, and smash it home."
-Megan Rapinoe

When I look back on my first year of teaching yoga, I see three mistakes which eventually solidified into three important lessons and remain my benchmarks for staying on track. Because they require daily devotion and cultivation, I call them the three essential mindsets: hard work, service, and authenticity.

First, when I graduated from teacher training, I underestimated the hard work ahead. Of course, I recognized that experienced teachers were better at teaching than me; I just didn't realize the amount of focus, consistency, and discipline it takes to get on their level. Great teachers make it look effortless, but it's not. Dolly Parton said, "It takes a lot of money to look this cheap," and just so with teaching yoga.

Behind every hour of skillful, instinctive instruction lie many hours of work—creating class plans until sequencing principles are in your bones, whittling your instructions down to eliminate all clutter, polishing cues until they are vivid and clear, devoting yourself to practicing with teachers who are better than you, and maintaining a healthy appetite to learn, learn, learn.

Most essential, though, is the hard work of teaching actual yoga classes to real people. Inevitably, in some of these actual classes, you will mess up. You will mess up in front of those real people. Or you will teach a class that, for whatever reason, is simply not good. When this happens, you will feel your stomach sinking, and you will believe everyone in the class hates you. After class, you will want to run out of the room and hide in the closet. It will feel bad. But I promise, the people don't hate you, and the class wasn't as bad as you think. I also promise you that it is completely normal to screw up when you are new at something. That's part of it: you make mistakes. Then you learn from your mistakes, put your head down, and get back to work. One day you look up, and you are better than before!

The second essential mindset is service. When I graduated from teacher training, I was more focused on myself than on serving my students. What I mean is that I was preoccupied with what students thought of me—whether they liked me—instead of learning to stand on my own approval by getting clear about what I wanted to offer people, and then doing my best to deliver it. I was putting my energy toward pleasing, instead of serving. The distinction here is subtle yet crucial, and it is palpable. Students can sense your energy, so it's important to keep your intentions clear and your mind in the right place. If you show up for class nervous or desperate to receive approval, people feel that. If you show up from a place of integrity with the intention to give your best, they feel that, too.

The third mindset is authenticity. I wasn't myself; I wasn't authentic. When I taught a class, it was almost like I went into character. In hindsight, I see what was happening: I didn't feel like I was a real yoga teacher, so it felt inappropriate to show up as myself. Instead, I adopted a persona. I spoke in a sing-song because I thought my regular voice sounded too suburban. I repeated things that I had heard other teachers say—cliches about opening the heart and constant reminders to "just breathe"—instead of speaking from my own heart and experience, and saying things I actually wanted to share with students.

I don't blame myself or regret it, though, because I believe that feeling like an imposter is a natural phase of development when you start a new job. In any case, I moved through the phase as I continued teaching and gradually gained confidence as an instructor. With more confidence, I opened up—speaking naturally, making jokes, and connecting with my students. If you are going through this phase right now, be patient with yourself, and remember that authenticity, including your imperfection, is magnetic.

For me, these three lessons in hard work, service, and authenticity are hard-won, and the struggle continues. I still have days when I feel like a total imposter. Sometimes I am exhausted and totally uninspired, and sick of yoga. The last thing I want to do is sit down with my notebook and plan classes for the week. When students are not picking up what I'm throwing down, it is not fun, and I fight my people-pleasing reflex to change my plan to satisfy a couple of tough customers. All this to say, teaching yoga is not an easy job, but it is worth it. Let's explore how these three habits can make what is difficult about the job manageable and rewarding.

Hard Work: No Shortcuts to Mastery

To be a good yoga teacher, you have to teach lots of yoga classes. Frequently, I see YTT graduates convince themselves that aren't ready to start teaching, in any context. They put off the inevitable by telling themselves that they need one more month of preparation, one more online anatomy course, one more year of taking classes, even a 300-hour certification, and *then* they will be ready. But in reality, if you wait to start teaching until you feel 100 percent ready, you will never start teaching. You simply have to jump in, ready or not.

The good news is you can start small by teaching in low-pressure environments. Volunteer, teach your friends, or start a donation-based class. In this way, you can make it feel more like wading in, rather than jumping. In Chapter 4, we will talk specifically about how to get started. For now, fortify yourself with the knowledge that every time you plan, teach, and reflect on a class, you get a little better. Literally, the "yoga teaching" part of your brain will blossom, like how London cab drivers have above-average hippocampi from constantly calculating routes in the crazy tangle of the city's streets.

The magic—the blossoming—happens when you approach each and every class you teach as an opportunity to learn and improve. I am a fan of selecting two skills you want to improve—for example, sequencing and vocal tone—and focusing on them for a couple of months. The more specific, the better. I guarantee that you will notice an improvement.

Right now, I'm focusing on giving three good adjustments and weaving a strong, authentic theme into every class. I draw a little heart next to the class in my planner when I meet my goals. But you have to master one set of skills to move onto the next. As you are starting out, you might focus simply on creating a class plan and making eye contact with your students. Once you have that down, you can progress into more nuanced aspects of teaching yoga.

Another practice I like to use is journaling after classes about what went well, and what could improve. I also write down questions that come up—things I realize I don't know—like how to modify for a pregnant woman in a Vinyasa class, or why a student might be having pain in a particular pose. Take five minutes after class and write using the Post-Class Reflection Template in the Resources section of the book.

Journaling helps me find clarity, track my progress, and stay motivated. But I have learned it is important to write more for "What Went Well" than "What to Improve." Otherwise, I fixate on little failures, and I get in a mindset of never good enough. I went through a phase like that recently where I could not stop beating myself up for things that students probably didn't notice, like not weaving my theme back into the class at its peak, or letting my vocal inflection creep up at the end of sentences.

If you use the journaling technique, approach it with a spirit of curiosity and a mindset of growth. Write down more positive things than negative, think of the negatives as opportunities to improve, and be nice to yourself. Also, remember that the people in your yoga classes are *way* more focused on themselves than on you. Unlike you, they are not journaling after every class about what you could have done better. They just want to move and breathe, and they probably think you are doing just fine.

Here is another benefit of teaching lots of yoga classes: it will help you get a job. If you start teaching to your friends, family, church group, or strangers in a park, the experience can get you hired at studios and fitness centers—where they pay you! Studio Directors do not often hire applicants fresh out of teacher training. But people who have taught for a year—even just once per week or as a volunteer—are much more likely to get a callback to come in and demo.

Myself, I don't think I would have been hired at my studio without a year of teaching experience on my resumé when I applied. Never mind that it was a year during which I earned no money, my classes were tiny, and (as we already established) my emotions were unstable. It didn't matter. I listed three weekly classes on my resume, which got me in the door to give a demo class at a good studio. Then, during the demo itself, I was, in fact, a better teacher than I had been a year before because I had been practicing, failing, and learning. My point is, hard work is the way forward.

Service: It's Not About You

You already know that intention matters. You know that the mindset with which you approach a situation makes a big, if subtle, difference. For example, if your partner is having a difficult time at work, or a bout of depression, or a painful patch with a family member, and they talk to you about it, you can listen with the intention either to fix the problem or to support the person.

Fixing comes from distrust and fear. Fixing says you don't believe that your partner can handle it, and also that you are afraid of the discomfort, difficulty, and pain that the situation could bring into your lives. On the other hand, supporting comes from trust and love. You trust your partner to work through it, you give help out of love if they ask you for it, and you are strong enough to tolerate the uncomfortable feelings that arise without pushing them away.

When it comes to yoga teaching, there are two similar mindsets. The first is based on ego and fear. In this mindset, your focus is on getting approval, praise, and pleasing people. The second mindset is based on service and love. In this mindset, your focus is on serving your students the best you can, according to your values and mission statement as a teacher, which we will cover in the next chapter.

Similar to the difference between fixing and supporting, the difference between pleasing and serving is subtle. Serving your students does not mean making everyone happy all the time—and thank God because that is impossible, and you will drive yourself crazy if that is your measure of success. "Yoga" means different things to different people, and everyone has different preferences. Inevitably you will have students that do not like your particular style of teaching. Service means getting clear on what you want to offer people and deliver it with integrity.

Even as I write this, I know that I slip into the first mindset of trying to win approval when I'm not feeling confident, when I am overstressed, and when I am disconnected from my own practice. Basically, when I'm not grounded, I start hustling to impress people—to prove my worth—instead of focusing on my job. I make the yoga class all about me instead of my students.

For example, a few weeks ago my friend Jill popped into my regular Tuesday night Vinyasa class. Jill is like a cool older sister to me. She plays the harmonium and teaches Bhakti. She is really smart, and a badass, and full of love. I respect her a lot, and her opinion matters to me. When I saw her walking up to the studio, I panicked because on that particular day I didn't have time to plan class. My plan was to teach something simple and make stuff up as I went (side note: sometimes that does work out great). But now, that plan felt dangerously inadequate. I thought I needed something impressive, unique, and complex with an amazing theme to prove to Jill that I was a good teacher.

So, in the five minutes before class started, I scribbled some notes of what I could teach that might impress her, recycling a sequence from the week before, and I started class, all up in my own head. Preoccupied and nervous, I couldn't really be present with everyone else in the room.

I couldn't speak from my heart. And despite my desire to make the class a great one, it was not.

As students, I think we have all experienced the difference between a teacher who is open and present in class—giving off an energy of love—and one who is tense and distant—giving off an energy of fear. As a teacher, my worst classes happen when I'm in my head, wrapped up in fear of being judged and focusing on what my students think of me, instead of what I am passionate about offering. The best classes I teach are when I teach from my heart with the intention to serve my students through yoga.

When you feel yourself drifting toward fear, come back to service. Pause for a moment. Go into the bathroom if you need to be alone. Take a few deep breaths. Remind yourself what yoga means to you. What do you want to provide for your students? Maybe the answer is using deliberate breathing and movement to create an environment where people can explore the inner landscape, focus on the present moment, and experience increasingly subtle layers of reality all the way to the Divine. Or whatever. I don't know. Whatever it is for you, teaching yoga is not about proving something. It's not about you, it's about them.

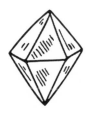

Authenticity: Be Yourself

Maybe "be yourself" sounds like a lesson that Hannah Montana learned at the end of an episode, or maybe every episode, but hear me out. Learning how to be yourself leading a yoga class, how to speak authentically, and how to connect with your students as people is essential to teaching great classes. Without a real connection, your teaching will feel hollow, and real connection requires authenticity.

As I wrote earlier, when I started teaching, I didn't feel like a real yoga teacher. As a result, I subconsciously believed that being myself in class by speaking in my regular voice and revealing my weird sense of humor would expose me as a fraud to my students. It would slowly dawn on them, "Hold on, she's not a real yoga teacher after all! She's just a person!" To prevent this, I spoke in a yoga voice, I was very serious, and I acted like someone who never, ever ate pizza.

Feeling like an imposter is a natural phase in any new job, especially when you are leading or instructing other people. My friend Ashley Day who teaches high school art told me that during her first year she used to wonder if her "Ms. Day" teacher persona would ever start to feel like her real self. She did, she said, after a year or two. Ashley and I talked about how it is hard to "be yourself" when you are stepping into a role that is new and challenging, one which you are scared you cannot fill. It is less scary, less vulnerable, to perform the role of a yoga teacher, based on some ideal in your head.

Gaining authenticity as a yoga instructor, then, is a gradual process. To move toward it with more grace and confidence, practice the first two habits in this chapter. Teach classes, even if you feel insecure, scared, and unprepared. The more you teach, the more you will improve. The more you improve, the more you will authentically feel like a good teacher. When you really feel like a good teacher, you'll be comfortable acting like yourself in class. And that's when the real magic can flow.

In the meantime, take a few deep breaths before each class. Remind yourself why you want to teach yoga in the first place, and of the benefits you want people to receive. Try to speak to your class as individuals who are there to practice and learn yoga, not to judge you. One of my teachers says that you actually don't need to be more advanced physically, spiritually, or mentally to be a yoga teacher. Rather, your job is to provide time and space for people to practice. So take some pressure off yourself, and get out there.

You Can Do It!

Stepping into your new role as a yoga teacher is intimidating. Of course, it's also exciting, empowering, and fulfilling. But in your earliest days, the scale usually tips more toward scary than toward fun. When you find yourself feeling anxious or overwhelmed, remember that it is normal to feel that way. It's normal to struggle. It's supposed to be hard. This is a challenging job, and don't let people tell you otherwise!

I bet that every single one of your yoga teachers, who make it look so easy, felt like you do right now at some point. The only reason they are great at it now is that they got past their insecurities and they kept practicing. They forged ahead through nerves, messy classes, and self-doubt. They worked hard, every day and every class, to confront their fears and hone their craft. That's what you have to do now. Get out of your own head. Put in the hours of hard work. Focus on serving your students instead of worrying about what they think of you. And be yourself! Connect with people! It's just yoga!

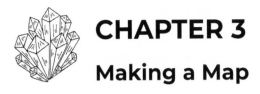

CHAPTER 3

Making a Map

"A vision without a task is a dream. A task without a vision is drudgery. But a vision with a task can change the world."

–Black Elk

After you graduate yoga teacher training, start teaching yoga—to your friends, for your mom, for free, at the park, in the dark, in a tree, in a box, with a fox! That was a silly way to deliver a serious piece of advice, but I am serious. When you plan, rehearse and teach classes regularly, you become exponentially more comfortable and skilled at teaching yoga, in less time than you might think. The neural pathways in your brain deepen, and the yoga section of your brain grows more robust.

Earlier in my teaching career, I used to go to sleep at night and dream that I was instructing a class. Nothing weird or surreal happened in these dream classes. I wasn't naked or toothless or riding a whale or anything. I was literally just teaching regular, straightforward classes. A little boring? Yes. But also amazing? Heck yes! My brain was forming new connections so fast! Recently, my yoga dreams returned when I was intensely focused on learning a new sequencing method.

I know this happens to other people too. During one module of my 300-hour training at Kripalu Center for Yoga and Health, I stayed in the dorm rooms with about 16 other women in the program. A few nights into the training, one of my roommates was talking in her sleep, which woke us up. At first, no one could make out what she was saying, but then someone said, "I think she's teaching Warrior II." Listening closer, she was indeed. Someone said it would be funny if we were circled around her bed in Warrior II when she woke up, but it was late so we went back to sleep instead. For the best—that would have been terrifying for her.

Anyway, your brain is amazing, and when you start putting what you learned into practice, you will blossom. Yet, along with the growth spurt, you will also experience rough patches—times when you feel like you are making no progress at all. You will doubt yourself. Your confidence will droop and your motivation will lag.

It feels gross, and it's not limited to new teachers. In fact, I'm having a rough week right now, as I write this. I feel like I'm not connecting with my students, like there's a barrier between what I really want to say and what actually comes out of my mouth. My classes feel stale to me. I'm wondering if I even actually understand the fundamentals of good sequencing, if I even know how to teach a decent class! Last night, going to bed, I told Dan, "I know this is an old, boring story of mine, but I felt like everyone hated my class today." It's such a familiar phase of a cycle at this point that he didn't even indulge me, "Jack, you know that's not true." And I do know that. By next week, I will feel much better, partly because that's how the cycle goes, and partly because I have a tool to help me get back on track.

That tool is a mental map. During this current rough patch, instead of staying stuck in the swamp of self-doubt and unable to see the path out, my map helps me put the swamp in the context of a whole landscape. It helps me remember that it's not all swamp. I'm just having a bad week, but I know what I'm working toward, and I know why I am doing it. I know where to focus, and how to pull myself out of the mud.

When you are embarking on anything challenging and new, a map is helpful. It tells you where you are now, where you want to go, and the steps you can take every day to get closer to it. A map gives you the big picture, as well as the daily steps forward.

As a new yoga teacher, you can make your map in three layers. Start with sketching the landscape, which illustrates your purpose and describes why you teach. Next, plot your destination, which marks the goals you are moving toward. Finally, trace the path to get there—the daily tasks and best practices that will gradually bring you closer to your destination. Together these three elements—landscape, destination, and path—create a mental map that will help keep you motivated and connected to your purpose, even during bad weeks.

1. **Landscape:** the big picture, why you teach, your mission statement
2. **Destination:** your goals, your dream job, your definition of success
3. **Path:** the small, daily steps that move you forward

Landscape: The Big Picture, Why You Teach, Your Mission Statement

The first layer of your map is the big picture: what yoga means to you and why you want to be a teacher. These questions are huge, and the answers change, so don't pressure yourself to have complete, definitive, life-long answers right now. Instead, start where you are. Like an explorer in new territory, you will fill out sections of the landscape as you discover more about yourself and your practice over many years. For now, start where you are. Get out a pen and paper and spend 20 minutes writing stream-of-consciousness answers to the following questions. Then use your answers to create a mission statement you read every day or before each every class.

Sketching Your Mission Statement

- What's the point of yoga?
- What are your core values?
- How do you hope people feel after class?
- Why are you a yoga teacher?
- What is the role of a yoga teacher?
- Which aspects of yoga are you most excited to share?
- In teaching, what does your best effort look like?
- What are your best qualities as a human?
- Describe a great yoga class in three words.
- What do you hope people say about your classes?

I feel a huge difference between the times when I feel grounded in my mission and when I do not. I have revised it a few times over the years. Here is one I wrote a couple of years ago.

> *Devoted to excellence, but kind toward my shortcomings, I strive to teach yoga classes that help my students feel grounded, alive, balanced, and healthy. I work every day toward this goal by showing up in service to my students rather than my own ego, preparing for each and every class, leading by example by "living my yoga," and being present and authentic with people.*

And here is a more recent version, which is more like a prayer. Right now, I love it. It is just right for where I am today. But maybe in a year I will think it's super melodramatic.

> *My job is to give people time and space for their practice. My job is to help people feel healthy, confident, and comfortable in their bodies. My job is to lead a fun and nourishing practice of movement, breathing, and contemplation that helps people cultivate a rich and tangible spirituality every day. May the result be a world with more love, more clarity, and more faith. May the result be stronger families and communities. May the result be less separation and alienation from each other. May I be present, connected, and authentic. May I speak from my heart. May I do my best, earn their trust, and give something of value. May I not take myself too seriously.*

Destination: Your Goals, Your Dream Job, What Success Means

A couple of years ago, Dan and I took a trip to Olympic National Park, and spent a week camping in the backcountry. It was gorgeous: tiers of dark green pines, autumn wildflowers, high ridges overlooking blue mountains. Every afternoon, we picked enough wild blueberries to fill our quart-sized Nalgene bottles and ate them with oatmeal for breakfast in the morning. By the way, if the apocalypse happens and I survive to join a ragtag group of travelers, I want my job to be berry-gatherer.

But it was also so hard! The trails were steep and the switchbacks endless. My shoulders ached from my 40-pound backpack that didn't fit my body quite right. My knees killed. Black bears meandered around the trails, and although they were clearly much more interested in eating the blueberries than my meaty little calves, I still felt pinpricks of fear every time we rounded a bend. Worst of all, there was no pizza! By day two, I was daydreaming about the end of the trip, when we could soak in the hot springs at the park lodge, and there would be pizza.

Running parallel to my fantasies of modern American pleasures was irritation with myself. I had been looking forward to this trip for months! Getting here took a lot of planning and effort. Simply getting to the trailhead was a long ordeal: 5 a.m. flight from St. Louis to Seattle, a train from the airport to the city, a bus out of Seattle, a transfer to another bus toward the peninsula, then hitchhiking into the park itself. After all that, it felt ridiculous to wish it was over. I needed to fix my attitude.

As a yogi, I wish I could tell you that I just remembered to be mindful, and everything was okay, but that's not what happened. For sure, my yoga training did help. For example, I practiced feeling the sensation of craving pizza in my body and letting it pass without pushing it away, exactly like the *sramanas* of yore. But actually, what helped was asking Dan to hand over the map eight times a day, and breaking the trip down into small sections.

After I did that, I could relax into the whole experience—the good parts and the hard parts. I could see how each section of steep trail was bringing me closer to the mountaintop or an alpine lake, and how each day's efforts brought us closer to the warm and cozy lodge, and indeed, to pizza. When I felt connected to our purpose and progress, I could enjoy myself instead of wishing it was over. I could simultaneously be content where I was and see how it fit into reaching our destination.

Similarly, I have a vision of the amazing yoga teacher I'll be in five, ten, and 20 years from now. In the future, my classes are reliably inspiring, relatable, fresh, fun, and deeply healthful. I am great at hands-on assists and adjustments. I have a strong presence, charisma, and magnetism. I am teaching all sorts of interesting and diverse workshops, retreats, and courses. I am eating pizza in the lodge.

With that destination on my map, I can focus on how each class can bring me closer to my goals, even during weeks when I'm feeling low. I can appreciate where I am today—the victories and the hard work—instead of believing I'll only be happy and satisfied when I reach some idea of an ultimate goal.

Healthy goal-setting means taking time to figure out what real, authentic success means to you, based on your deep values. Then you have to align your daily work toward that goal. As you move toward it, try to enjoy where you are on the path every day. Don't just wish for it to be over and believe that you can't be happy until you achieve your goals. Do you already have specific goals? If so, write them down. If not, here are some questions to help you figure it out. Spend some time journaling on them, and then write three or four clear vision sentences to describe your thoughts. An example is below.

Plot Your Destination

- Do you want teaching yoga to be your only job, a part-time job, or an "honored hobby?"
- What type of classes (big groups, small groups, privates) do you enjoy teaching the most?
- How many classes per week do you want to teach?
- Do you want to work for yourself, like an independent contractor at many different places, or as part of a team, employed at one studio?
- How much income do you need to support the life you want?

- Identify any special interests, such as prenatal yoga, yoga for trauma, yoga for youth, restorative yoga, yoga in the workplace.
- Write out a day-in-the-life of your dream job. Be as specific as possible.

You can have multiple destinations for the near, medium and long-term. Here's an example of a destination that a new yoga teacher might have for three years down the road.

In three years, I am working full-time as a yoga teacher, teaching eight to ten group yoga classes and three to four private lessons per week. I teach from a place of service to my students, and I feel like most classes connect with my students. I give skillful hands-on adjustments. I have an email list of at least 100 students that I can use to market my offerings, and I'm planning to lead a yoga retreat in the next year.

Path: The Small, Daily Steps That Move You Forward

The top layer of your map is the path, which winds through your landscape toward your destination. Like campsites, your path is a series of small daily accomplishments that approach your goal. Tracing your path is simple. Make a list of ten small steps you can take toward your destination and deadlines. Make them as specific as possible. Do them. Rest. Breathe. Then make another list. Repeat.

Take the destination example above—working full-time as a yoga teacher three years from now—some steps in your path for the first couple months might include:

Charting Your Path

1. *Purchase liability insurance.*
2. *Spend 30 minutes brainstorming places to volunteer to teach.*
3. *Contact three places from the list.*
4. *Email friends and family to let them know I completed my training and I am looking for opportunities to get experience.*
5. *Organize one class in the park on Sunday for family and friends.*
6. *Find a class taught by a potential mentor teacher to attend regularly.*
7. *See if Dad wants to do an eight-week private yoga session to improve flexibility and breathing to practice working with clients one-on-one.*
8. *Have coffee with Melissa, who teaches at the studio where I want to work.*
9. *Continue personal practice, 30 minutes in the morning.*
10. *Contact the owner of Studio A to ask about sub list.*

Without a Map, You Will Get Lost

If you start working and you haven't taken the time to sit down and make a map of what you really want, you will move toward something, but it might not be the *right* thing. When I first started teaching yoga, Dan and I had recently moved to New England for his job, where we didn't know anyone. I taught classes independently, so I didn't have a real-life yoga community of mentors and peers as examples of healthy, normal careers. By default, I looked to the most visible example of success I saw: yoga celebrities. Without consciously choosing it, fame became my definition of success.

I pursued that definition of success with some enthusiasm for a brief time, but it did not feel right. Gradually, I realized I didn't want to be famous, I just hadn't taken the time to figure out my other options. I didn't want to put my energy into building an online presence, and I definitely didn't want to prowl for Twitter followers. I wanted to teach in-person classes and have co-workers. I wanted to be part of a community, to feel valued, to ride my bike to work, to have time for fun and exploration, and to earn a middle-class income. Once I came to that realization, sat down and mapped out a different future, my work felt satisfying and aligned with my values.

We live in a culture that tells us that if we aren't doing something extremely special — if we are simply leading ordinary lives — we aren't doing something meaningful. That's a big burden to carry. But we don't have to accept it. Instead, we can be countercultural, and live by this Brené Brown motto: "Ordinary does not equal meaningless." That sentence is so soothing to me because it reminds me that to be successful, you do not have to go big. You do not have to be famous. You do not have to be the best. You do not have to earn praise from everyone all of the time. An ordinary, authentic life lived through service, gratitude, and love is very meaningful.

I hope this quote brings you comfort too. Keep it in mind when you are setting your goals. If the best way you can serve people and feel fulfilled is to teach one class a week while keeping your regular job at an office, don't feel like you aren't a "real" yoga teacher. If your classes are small, especially at first, that doesn't make them any less meaningful. Give your best to the people who *are* there. If the yoga practices you love to teach are simple and gentle, teach them from your heart and don't feel like you need to force some crazy arm balances into the sequence.

To be clear: I'm not saying that you shouldn't work hard to be the best possible instructor and to challenge yourself to do things that scare you. "Ordinary is meaningful" isn't an excuse to be complacent or avoid things that scare you. Don't settle for only teaching yoga to your parents if what you *really* want is to work at your favorite studio and lead retreats. Just don't get trapped in the celebrity-culture mindset that if you aren't extraordinary, then you aren't enough. Your best is always more than good enough.

Six Types of Yoga Careers

Here's some kindling to get your goal-setting fire burning. There are lots of models for how you can be a yoga teacher, from teaching full time to tending one class per week. You don't have to quit your desk job and only teach yoga, especially if you actually *like* your desk job. On the other hand, if you hate working in corporate America and what you *really* want is to teach yoga, you can find a way to make it happen. Start considering the different possibilities and find one that suits you.

The Yoga Hobbyist

Mark Stephens, the author of classic yoga texts including *Teaching Yoga* and *Yoga Sequencing*, describes how some people teach a couple of classes per week and for them teaching yoga is an "honored hobby." I love that phrase. Sometimes there's the idea that if it isn't your full-time job, then you're not as committed to it as someone who teaches 20 classes per week, but I don't believe that is true. Some of the most creative and committed teachers I know teach one or two awesome classes, week after week. If quitting your regular job isn't an option, know that you can still serve people so very well.

The Part-Time Yoga Teacher

Teaching yoga doesn't pay much—at least not for new teachers. If you want to support yourself solely on yoga money, you will be teaching a ton of classes at different places, which can be draining, especially when you are new and spending lots of time planning classes. That's why many teachers have part-time work that they can fit around their weekly teaching schedule. Maybe for you, the part-time job is temporary, a way to make ends meet while you build enough group classes and private lessons to eventually quit your

part-time job. Or maybe part-time teaching is a
long-term plan because you discover there is a
limit to the number of yoga classes you can teach
per week and still enjoy it. Either way, having a
non-yoga part-time job can be really supportive
and complimentary. It's healthy for your body to
move and exercise in new and diverse ways, and
it's healthy for your mind to earn income in new
and diverse ways too.

The Yoga Teacher/Therapist

A tried and true career combination is teaching yoga and being a certified therapist in another field: a massage therapist, craniosacral therapist, hypnotherapist, doula, Thai bodyworker,
mental health counselor, psychotherapist, and
many more options ranging from the traditional
to the new age. In fact, some of the most prom-
inent yoga and meditation teachers have a background in therapy, including Tara Brach and
Stephen Cope. Principles in therapy and in yoga
often overlap, and many therapists use yoga
methods to help their clients.

The Full-Time Instructor

Another option is to teach yoga full time. If
that sounds like an ideal situation to you, I am
excited for you to start working toward it! Just
know that it can take a while to accumulate
enough classes at decent pay rates to make it
work, financially and physically. Compensation is
usually lower for new teachers, which means you
could end up teaching an insane number of

classes per week, and burning out. Have patience, practice exquisite self-care, and look for the higher paying gigs like private clients. Experience counts toward higher pay at gyms and studios, as do class sizes. There's no shortcut—just years of focused, consistent work.

The Online Teacher

Teaching yoga online helps you bring yoga to a wider audience, including people who don't have access to a yoga studio due to location, cost, or physical limitations. I love that there are so many high-quality yoga classes on YouTube because it is free, private, and customizable for anyone who wants it. Yes, there's a lot of competition, but there is always room for an authentic voice. Very popular hosts can make a good full-time income from YouTube. You need high production quality to be one of those people and a big portfolio of work, but don't be discouraged if you don't have access to set lighting and a good camera right now. Use your iPhone or whatever you have and start building a collection of videos.

The Yoga Celebrity

I'm talking about people such as Seane Corn, Kathryn Budig, Shiva Rae, and Rodney Yee—yogis who make a good living leading international retreats, headlining yoga conferences, writing books, and producing online yoga courses. If becoming a top world-famous teacher is your dream, there's no reason you can't get there with the right connections, business savvy, and years of devotion. A good friend who studies with a nationally known teacher told me that he said to her, "There are lots of yoga teachers out there, but there's also a lot of room at the top." If you want to be at the top of the field, go for it! Just make sure you stay clear on your motivations.

Writing Your Yoga Teacher Bio

The first time I attempted a yoga bio I spent about two hours writing six sentences. I had just finished my 200-hour training and had yet to teach a real class. As I struggled to describe myself, I realized it is hard to write a professional bio when you have no professional experience. Imagine that! Also, it's weird to write about yourself in the third person. You feel like Elmo. When I finally finished, though, I was happy with the result. Or, maybe simply delirious from typing, deleting, and rewriting flattering statements about myself all afternoon.

A year later I reread it and physically cringed. The tone was cheeky and inauthentic. I deleted the whole thing and wrote it again. And when I reread *that* one a few months later, I didn't like it either! Five years later, I have a bio on a studio website at this very moment that I do not like and have been meaning to edit.

Bios are weird and no matter how long you spend on one, you are never going to make it perfect. It's something that you will always be revising because you yourself are always changing. Over time, you will clarify your teaching style and your understanding of what you offer. You will find better ways to describe yourself, and more experience to include in your bio.

So, don't agonize over your first attempt like I did. Instead, keep it simple, use a light touch, knowing you will probably completely rewrite it sometime soon. Set a timer for 30 minutes and write five to seven sentences that answer the questions below. Then proofread it, ask someone else to proof it, and let it go until it's time to update it.

Prompts for Writing Your Bio

- Where did you complete your 200-hour training?
- What styles of yoga do you teach?
- What's your yoga story? When and how did you start practicing? Keep this brief.
- What do you hope your students get out of your class? How do you hope they feel afterward?
- Do you have any other specialized training or experience that relates to yoga?
- Say a little something about your personal life: what do you like to do in your free time?
- How can people contact you?

You Can Do It!

Whatever your map looks like, wherever you want to go, however nervous or scared or excited you feel about the journey, I am here to tell you that you can do it. One step at a time, you can become the teacher you are meant to be. With many days of practice, devotion, and passion, you can reach your full potential: you can be a really good yoga teacher! You can make a positive difference in people's lives. You can have a job that makes you excited and grateful, and you can do work that is meaningful and integrated into your spirituality and personal development.

But it takes courage, patience, and tenacity. It also takes passion, but you already have that, right? No one decides to teach yoga for the money or job security. You fell in love with yoga for a reason. You signed up for teacher training for a reason. You got this book for a reason. You have a spark inside of you. Don't let it die by because you are scared of failing or being exposed or not being good enough. Work through that part. Use it as fuel. Have faith that you will come out on the other side. Most importantly, get ready to work. That's up next.

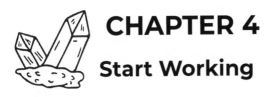

CHAPTER 4
Start Working

"Great people do things before they are ready."

-Amy Poehler

Taking that next step of teaching actual yoga classes out in the world can feel more like a giant leap than a "next step," and many people delay it, or worse, never take it.

Putting yourself in front of people and calling yourself a yoga teacher for the first time is like jumping off the high dive into the pool: it's a gradual process until it's not. You step up the ladder, you walk down the diving board, then at some point you just have to step off and fall 33 feet to the water.

For another thing, even if you *are* psyched to cannonball into the pool, it can be hard to find work, especially work that pays. Most studios prefer to hire experienced teachers over teachers fresh out of YTT. This creates a situation where you can't get experience until someone hires you, but they won't hire you until you have the experience. It's a Catch-22 that can leave you stuck between a trainee and a teacher, not knowing how to move forward after you complete your program.

But it doesn't have to be that way. In this chapter, we will explore six routes to get unstuck—ways you can gain teaching experience in low-pressure environments while building your confidence, skills, and resume. After a year of that, you will be ready to reapply to studios.

The caveat is that you won't earn much money at first. During the year after my teacher training, I taught more than 250 classes for which I got paid little or nothing. I volunteered at a non-profit, rented studio space, and taught a donation-based class in what was basically an attic. As you know, many of those classes were not great. But they were so valuable. I needed that year of practice teaching to get to the next step of teaching at a studio, and I am grateful to the students who stuck with me.

In the yoga world, there are no internships to help bridge the gap between YTT and professional-level teaching. Some studios train their own teachers and have systems in place to phase them onto the staff, but that's the exception. More commonly, trainees come out the other side of YTT without a clear route toward a good career teaching yoga, after having spent thousands of dollars on the program. If you are serious about becoming a yoga teacher, oftentimes you have to create your own internship. That's what this chapter is about: creating your own path. Let's explore some possibilities and brainstorm ways that you can start working right now.

Route #1: Volunteer

You could volunteer! A great way to get experience is to volunteer at places where they don't have the budget to hire a yoga teacher, including nonprofits, community centers, and schools. Volunteering outside of the studio or gym setting has a few advantages. First, it's low pressure. At studios, students have expectations, preferences, and favorite teachers. Plus, they are paying for it. But when you volunteer, people are usually more open, with fewer expectations and less experience with yoga. Second, it's great practice. You will learn how to teach people who are brand new to yoga, have varying abilities, and possibly limited mobility. Third, you get to teach people who may not otherwise have access to yoga.

Over the years, I have volunteered at a halfway house, a refugee resettlement nonprofit, a gym for people with disabilities, a summer camp for kids, and a few other places. The summer after teacher training, I taught a free yoga class at my community garden on Saturday mornings. A small group of us would gather in an open patch before the sun got too hot for an hour of gentle yoga. The whole scenario was so pleasant that it was okay if my teaching wasn't perfect. After class, we worked in the plot where we grew food for a soup kitchen.

Sit down and brainstorm organizations in your community that you would like to support. Are there organizations that could benefit from yoga classes—to improve quality of life, collect donations, incentivize participation, or build community—but don't have the budget to hire a teacher? Think about the causes that you support. Ask family members or friends who work for nonprofits if they are interested. Send out an email; post on Facebook.

Here's the tricky part, though. Often, the people you teach as a volunteer in order to gain experience are the very people who would greatly benefit from a teacher who already has lots of experience because they have health issues, limited mobility, or lack of experience with yoga.

The same summer I taught garden classes, I also taught the class I mentioned earlier at a nonprofit gym for adults with disabilities, including some with acute mental illness. I loved that class, but looking back, I was not qualified to teach it. Several of my students had PTSD, and I had no training in trauma-informed yoga. Others had injuries and physical limitations like severe arthritis that I had no clue how to handle. Plus, most were brand new to yoga, and I don't think I did a good job teaching the basics.

It's ironic: I have found it is much harder to teach a basics class to newbies than an advanced class to hardcore practitioners. Yet, it is often the new teachers who end up teaching the volunteer classes to inexperienced students.

That doesn't mean you shouldn't do it; volunteering provides great experience. Just be humble and clear-eyed enough to recognize what you don't know. Every time you realize that you don't know something, look it up. If you realize your instruction for Downdog isn't working, go home and find new cues. If you panic when a student can only do yoga in a chair, do your whole sequence in a chair until you figure out all the options for her. If you trained as a Vinyasa teacher and you start teaching elderly people, learn how to teach something gentler. Basically, serve your students as best you can where you're at today, and use every class as an opportunity to get better at your job.

Route #2: Friends and Family

You can teach classes to your friends and family! Offer a regular class—once a month or once a week—at your house, in a park, at your church, or wherever else feels friendly. Invite your extended social network, It's fun, it's casual, and you will be more relaxed and confident teaching people who already love you than you would be in front of strangers. You could make it a free event or ask for donations. Also, make sure you ask for feedback on your class from your most honest friend.

Route #3: On Your Own

You can do it on your own! As I said earlier, the catch-22 of teaching yoga is that most studios prefer to hire people with teaching experience, but you cannot get teaching experience unless someone will hire you first. In other words, it can be hard to *get* teaching experience unless you already *have* teaching experience. Volunteering is one way around the hurdle. Another is running your own classes for a while: rent the studio space, advertise the classes, charge money, do the whole thing yourself.

First, let's talk about the downside. Teaching classes on your own can be expensive and a lot more work than volunteering somewhere or working for a studio. You could actually lose money instead of earning it, and you will spend a lot of time and energy hanging flyers and advertising your classes. Class sizes might be small, and you don't get the benefit of learning from more experienced teachers as a part of a community like you would at a studio.

Still, teaching classes independently can be great. You don't have to depend on someone hiring you, and you have more freedom. You can decide what to call your class and choose how you teach it. At a studio, you usually get plugged into whatever class they need filled: if it's advanced Hatha, that's what you have to teach even if your style is a slow Vinyasa. Third, you will get experience in the business of yoga, and start building a student base. Finally, it's an excellent test kitchen when you can ask students for feedback and improve your skills as an instructor.

Renting Studio Space

Start by finding a place to teach your classes. The first studio I rented was beautiful, with huge windows, brick interior walls, warm lighting and shiny hardwood floors, and a five-minute walk from my house.

The rental price seemed reasonable at $30 for a 75-minute class, and I didn't look anywhere else to compare. I calculated that if I charged $10 for drop-ins and sold class cards for $70, and five to seven people showed up for class, I could make $20 to $30 each class. If ten people showed up I could make $70! What if 20 people came?! $170 freaking bucks!

Fast forward six months and I was barely breaking even. Sometimes I had a big night with 12 students, but half the people were using the "First Class Free" cards I had distributed liberally throughout town. More often, I had three or four regular students in class who paid the discounted $7 class card rate. Between the small class sizes, my low rate, and the free class cards, it was not easy to make money.

Still, I was teaching yoga! Looking back, I am proud of myself and appreciative of the people who bought my class cards and took a chance on me. I feel grateful for the handful of regular students who came every week, in particular one woman who told me that my class helped her through a difficult year. I had been so involved with my own difficulties that I kind of forgot about the impact that yoga can have on students. Also, I learned something about the business of teaching yoga, I became a better instructor, and I realized that in the future I wanted to work at a studio instead of on my own.

The second time that I rented studio space, it was a work-trade arrangement. As I mentioned, I cleaned the studio once per week in exchange for one hour of use. The class was donation-based, and I always took home $20 to $70 in cash. Dan helped me clean and together it took 20 minutes.

If you're reluctant about spending money to teach yoga, a work trade is a great way to get access to studio space without the cost. Check out unconventional places where you can get cheap, free, or bartered access to a spacious room, like a community center, church meeting hall, martial arts studio, or even a conference room.

Advertising Your Classes

For me, the worst part of teaching independently was advertising the classes. I didn't have any Facebook friends in the new town where I lived, and paid ads on Facebook weren't yet a thing. Actually, maybe they were, and I was just out of touch. In any case, I would ride my bike around to hang flyers at coffee shops and health food stores. I posted about it on Craigslist; got some creepy responses. And that was the extent of my marketing efforts.

Now I know more about promoting my stuff, online and in person. It also helps that we moved back to our hometown and I have, like, a *million* Facebook friends here, guys. Yes, I'm pretty cool. We will talk more about marketing in Chapter 9, and I will lay out a way to advertise in a way that is honest, effective, and integrated into what you offer. For now, consider the idea that your marketing should give something valuable to potential clients. When you post on Facebook, don't just put up a picture of you with prayer hands looking off into the distance. Instead, teach people something that will help them. Make a short video of a breathing technique, or tell them how to do a headstand and its benefits. You will build trust, credibility, and a client base this way. If people get something of value out of your content, they will feel compelled to come to learn from you in person.

Pricing Your Classes

Deciding how much to charge for your first classes is tricky. When I was trying to figure it out, I checked to see what the other yoga teacher charged who rented the same studio space. But she had 20 years experience and a ton of specialized training. I didn't feel right charging the same rate as her. Clearly, her classes were better than mine, and they were indeed worth more. But on the other hand, I didn't want to undervalue myself or make classes so cheap that people got suspicious, like when you are at a thrift store and see a half dozen of the same brand-new shirt and you think, "What's wrong with this shirt."

Ultimately, I set my prices about 30 percent lower than the average local studio. I couldn't compete with them on teacher experience, name recognition, reputation, or on the number of classes offered per week, but I could make it more affordable and attract the people who couldn't afford studio prices. At the same time, the price wasn't so low that I devalued myself.

When it comes to charging money, the key is balance. Be realistic about the level you're at while giving yourself credit. Since you *are* brand new, it may not be appropriate to charge top rates. Plus, if your classes cost the same or more than those at established studios, you won't tap the market of students looking for a more affordable option. At the same time, don't swing too far in the other direction and feel like you have to make your classes dirt cheap. You might be new at this, but you completed a 200-hour teacher training, dang it! You are sharing something valuable. You work hard, and you deserve to be compensated for your time and effort. A fair price balances the humility of a beginner with the confidence of someone who stands behind the quality of their classes.

Route #4: Gyms and Fitness Centers

You could work at a gym! Purely based on my own observations and not any kind of data (sorry!), I will tell you that fitness centers are often hiring, and they may be more likely than studios to hire newer teachers, making them a great place to get started. Sometimes yoga people look down at gym yoga classes because fitness is the focus, but the very first yoga classes I took were at gyms, and I got a lot beyond the physical practice. I often came away from classes at the 24-Hour Fitness feeling inspired and full of insight. It is definitely possible to teach fitness classes infused with spiritual teachings. That said, you should expect the classes to be more about working out than inner work. If you don't like teaching that way, you may not like working at a gym.

Route #5: Studios

I have said that most studios won't hire you if you don't have any teaching experience, but that's not true in all cases. For example, if you live somewhere where there aren't many teach-ers, you might find yourself in high demand. Or you might get lucky and email a studio owner on the very day that she is desperate to find a teacher to fill a class.

My point is it never hurts to ask. Go ahead and apply to studios, especially studios where you already practice or—even better—where you trained. You can ask about teaching a weekly class, getting on their sub list, or even working as reception staff. If they don't have a teaching job open, the latter two options are a great way to learn about the studio, get to know the staff and students, take lots of classes from their best teachers, and position yourself to become a regu-lar teacher when the time is right.

When I started applying to studios, I had a lot of questions. I wasn't sure how it would compare to applying for a retail or office job. What's the best way to contact a studio owner? Should my resumé look like a traditional resumé? Should I wear yoga clothes to the interview or a nice in-terview outfit? What type of questions would they ask me in the interview? What about teach-ing a demo class? If you have similar questions, I hope my experience will shed some light.

Contacting Studios

Before you contact a studio owner or manag-er, take a bunch of classes there. It will show your interest and commitment, and prepare you to sub those classes in the future. Also, you can meet the staff and ask for advice or an introduc-tion to the studio owner. I have found that it does not work well to cold email studio owners without having been to the studio. When I have tried, I have received friendly but brief replies encouraging me to come to class first, and then check back. In contrast, studio owners have been receptive and enthusiastic when I have been to classes there before asking about a job.

If you are reaching out via email, introduce yourself and include where you did your training, and the style of classes you teach. Don't make it long—two or three sentences is good. Next, describe what you like about the studio. Be specific—which classes, which teachers, which features of the space. Finally, directly ask for what you want—a teaching job, a slot on the sub list, a conversation, whatever it may be. Most studio owners are busy people, so the easier you can make it for them, the better. Also, note that many studios have job applications online. Check that first and submit the application before you contact a studio about a job so that you follow their hiring protocols.

Writing Your Resumé

I have written lots of resumes for lots of different jobs. I have massaged my work experience to fit everything from a promotional exam writer to farm assistant to freelance reporter to hardware store clerk. But when I sat down to write a yoga resume, I was at a loss.

I had two problems. First, I didn't think that I had enough yoga experience to fill a page, unless I used 48-point font to write "200-hour teacher training!" and "LOVES DOING YOGA." Second, I didn't know how to phrase the little experience teaching yoga I did have. I didn't know how to translate a non-traditional job into a traditional format. Should I use standard resumé jargon such as, "Successfully implemented stress-reduction tactics into group learning," or "Dynamically cultivated client-based functional movement strategies?" No, you say? Right.

After a few tries, though, I figured it out. For one, work experience doesn't have to be yoga experience. If you have experience in sales, put it down. Studio owners will like that because you will be able to sell memberships. If you have worked as a school teacher, camp counselor, tutor, or trainer, it means you know how to lead groups and plan lessons. If you have ever had a customer service job, you have people skills that overlap with studio work. At first, you might feel like you don't have enough to fill a resume, but keep thinking about it and I bet you do.

As for the problem of writing a resumé for a non-traditional job, it turned out not to be a problem at all, but actually kind of fun. It is freeing! You can be creative. Stick with the general format of a one-sheet resumé because it's easier to read, but let it reflect your personality. Include the following:

What To Include on Your Resumé

- ❧ An objective—a simple and clear statement on why you want to teach yoga at that studio
- ❧ A profile—similar to your bio, describe your teaching philosophy and style

- Your teacher training—list your 200-hour program, its philosophy, and key learnings
- Additional trainings—workshops, online courses, meditation classes, etc.
- Work experience teaching yoga—any classes you have taught, paid or unpaid
- Other relevant work experience

The Interview

Your interview with a studio owner or manager could be anything from a casual conversation in the studio, to a cup of coffee, to a more formal situation in an office. Regardless of the format, interviews are about getting a sense for you as a person and whether you could be a good fit. Specifically, the person doing the hiring is probably trying to get a sense of three main things:

1. **You know what you're doing.** Your instruction is good, your voice is clear, you are confident, and you have a good handle on the basics of teaching yoga.
2. **You will be a good fit at the studio.** Your personality is compatible with the studio, and you can teach the style of classes that they need you too.
3. **You are available when they need you.** The more classes you are able to teach, the better, especially if you are applying to be a sub.

That's general criteria. Now here are specific questions you might be asked. Practice with a friend so you have an idea for what you are going to say, but try not to sound rehearsed,

Interview Questions

- ☼ Tell me about your 200-hour training.
- ☼ What did you like most about your training? What do you think your 200-hour training lacked?
- ☼ Describe your teaching style.
- ☼ Describe your yoga practice.
- ☼ How would you modify an intermediate or advanced level class for a beginner student?
- ☼ Tell me about a time when you had to give special modifications or accommodations to a student.
- ☼ What type of classes are you most comfortable teaching?
- ☼ How did you hear about the studio?
- ☼ Why do you want to work here?
- ☼ What type of support do you want from us, as a studio?

A note on attire: unless you will be teaching a demo class conjoined to the interview, your best bet is to wear a professional, non-yoga outfit. Somewhere on the spectrum from pantsuit to yoga pants. Think Hillary Clinton attempting to seem laid back.

The Demo Class

Usually you will teach a demo class as part of the hiring process, which is stressful because your "students" will likely be the studio owner, managers, and teachers, all of whom have a lot more experience than you. I have also done a demo class where I subbed a regular class while the teacher evaluated me, which was equally stressful!

I participate in demo classes and help evaluate the teachers afterward, and from being on the other side what I have learned makes for a strong demo class.

1. **Be present and confident.** The most important thing about teaching a demo class is the energy you bring to it. Relax, smile, and make eye contact. Stand up straight. I know it's nerve-racking, but try to calm yourself enough to be friendly and present with the people you are teaching. Studios want to hire teachers who will connect with students, and when you're calm you will be more confident and capable.

2. **Have a theme.** A thoughtfully planned sequence shows that you know what you are doing. You could sequence to a peak pose, integrate a philosophical theme, or focus on a particular area of the body. While regular students may not pick up on your sequencing, the studio staff in your demo class will be thinking about what you are doing, why, and how it all fits together.

3. **Be conservative on the music.** In one demo that I evaluated, the instructor played Cat Stevens *the entire time,* which was distracting because I don't like Cat Stevens enough to listen to him for an hour, and neither do my

two coworkers who were also part of the demo. Plus, at our studio, teachers usually don't play music with lyrics. It was hard to focus on evaluating her teaching and to enjoy the class because I kept thinking, "I can't believe she's playing another Cat Stevens song!" Before you play music at a demo class, make sure it's appropriate and not distracting. If you aren't sure, ask before the demo.

4. **Start slow and calm.** It might be a good idea to start the class with a quiet, grounding meditation or gentle stretches. Even if you normally like to start with a bit more energy, consider a quieter start to your demo class, so that you can calm yourself down and make everyone else feel good too.

5. **Assume the best.** Usually the studio staff evaluating your demo class will understand if you seem a little nervous. Also, they know what it is like; they have all been in your position at some point. Assume the best: that they want you to do well, and they will be generous and forgiving of mistakes you might make because you are a little nervous.

6. **Focus on your intention, not the outcome.** I am glad to be writing this book for yoga teachers, who understand this concept better than the average bear. Of course, you want the outcome of your demo class to be getting hired. But if you focus on that, you turn the experience into a pass/fail test, and freak yourself out. If it's a test, you are worried about being judged, messing up, and not be-

ing good enough. Instead, focus on your intention—to do your best, serve your students, and learn from the experience no matter what. Make it an experience instead of a test, and your open, relaxed, and confident energy will radiate.

Route #6: Teaching Private Lessons

You could teach private lessons to friends and family for free, cheap, or trade! It's a good way to practice giving clear verbal instruction, adjustments, and working with different bodies. You will become a better teacher and when you apply for jobs, you can honestly say that you have been giving private yoga lessons for the past six months. I gave private lessons to my sister-in-law when she was pregnant for the first time, and it helped me learn about prenatal modifications and adjustments. Plus, it was nice to spend time together.

When it comes to informal private lessons, consistency is good. It provides structure, accountability, and a measure of progress to an arrangement that might otherwise devolve into an hour of chatting and lazy stretching. Schedule weekly sessions for a month or two. Ask your "client" about an issue they would like to address using yoga and do your research. Find some techniques and practices that could help, and then track the progress.

Farther down the road, when you have more experience, you can start charging real money. In fact, you can usually earn more per hour teaching private lessons compared to group classes. But first make sure that you are truly prepared to give a student their money's worth. Clients are willing to pay much more (often six times more) for a private lesson because they want something more specialized than they can get in a group class, like help recovering from an injury, deeper explanations of the poses, physical adjustments, or help with anxiety. So before someone shells out that kind of money for you, make sure you can really offer what they need.

Eight Tips for Getting Started

1. **Start small.** Don't expect yourself to hit the ground running teaching 20 classes each week. It takes time to pick up that many classes, and even if you could you would get overwhelmed and burned out. Focus on teaching one or two classes per week the best you can, and let your yoga career grow organically from there.

2. **Put out lots of fishing lines.** A good rule of thumb is that eight out of 10 ideas you have of places to teach won't work out. Either they won't be hiring, or it won't be a good fit, or you won't like it there, or the class won't work with your schedule. Make lots of connections, go out to do yoga at lots of places, and cultivate lots of relationships to gradually build a schedule that works for you.

3. **Don't limit yourself to gyms and studios.**
   You might be wondering, what if there aren't
   ten total studios where I live? As I said earlier,
   studios aren't the only place to get experience
   teaching. Expand your search to your kid's
   school, your office, your church, someone
   else's office, retreat centers, camps, retire-
   ment homes, local festivals, yoga clothing
   stores, etc. Same goes even if you live in a big
   city with lots of yoga studios.

4. **Be open to working without pay at first.** This
   is a bit controversial. People who disagree
   with me have a valid point: working for free
   can drives down pay for everyone else, deval-
   ue our profession, and sometimes take advantage of new teachers. But context matters.
   If you are volunteering to teach people who
   would not otherwise have access to yoga, you
   are not driving down wages for studio teachers. Sane for free classes for a fundraiser or a
   community event. I believe that, in the early
   days, the experience is valuable in itself.

5. **Follow up with contacts.** If a studio owner
   doesn't respond to your first email, don't assume that she read it, laughed at the idea of
   hiring you, and deleted it. Emails get buried,
   and people intend to respond and then forget. Always, always, always follow up with another email, another call, or three.

6. **Hire yourself.** If you're having no luck finding a job, you know who will *definitely* hire
   you? You! As we discussed, start teaching a
   class on your own at a park, your church, or

rented studio space. It can be a lot of work for little money, but it's experience and that's what counts right now.

7. **Collaborate with other teachers.** Yes, there are lots of yoga teachers out there, but there are also lots of people who want to learn yoga. The potential market is big and growing. We teachers don't have to see each other as competition. Support and collaborate with your peers by offering sincere encouragement, trading feedback, or practicing teaching skills together. Cooperation breeds more success than competition.

8. **Think about the big picture.** When you feel frustrated and not good at teaching yoga, pause and put the moment into context. Imagine the teacher you want to be five, ten, twenty years from now. What are your classes like? How does it feel to teach them? How does it impact people? What's it like to be masterful? Try to clearly imagine all of it. Then determine what you need to do to get there.

You Can Do It!

A few years ago, I emailed the director of a university recreation center to ask if they were hiring yoga teachers. He wrote back a short message to say that they were not, explaining, "Not only is yoga popular, but so is being an instructor." Rude! But true. There *are* a lot of yoga teachers in the world, and more people graduate from teacher training every month. As a result, competition for jobs can be tough, and because supply is greater than demand, pay is usually not great at first. You may need to put in years of hard work and practice before you have the job you imagined when you signed up for teacher training.

Please, don't get discouraged, though. Try to be patient, focused, and dedicated. Take it one day at a time—do your best one class at a time. Learn something new every day. Go to lots of classes. Keep your motivations in check. Stay the course. Becoming a great yoga teacher and finding a great work situation requires years of practicing, studying, serving, making connections, and building a good reputation. But the hardest part is getting started. Once you do, you start to gather momentum. You will be pushed forward by the satisfaction of improving at something you love. And you will gain the confidence of knowing that you can do it!

CHAPTER 5

Rising to Challenges

"Easy is overrated."

- Brené Brown

There is a book that I love called *Teaching People, Not Poses* by Jay Fields, who writes that she decided to become a teacher because she loved the way she felt after *taking* a yoga class, and she figured she would feel ten times better after *teaching* one. Until I read that, I hadn't realized that that was why I did teacher training, too. I wanted "more of this." I wanted my life to be centered on the feeling of practicing yoga.

In reality, teaching a satisfying yoga class is a totally different experience from taking a satisfying yoga class. When you are in the zone as a teacher, it does feel amazing, but in a different way than being in the zone as a student. Plus, that amazing feeling comes with a set of challenges that don't exist for yoga students. As an instructor, you have to work through feeling self-conscious, having stage fright, getting burnt out, managing student expectations, feeling uninspired, seeking approval, and more. It can be difficult and disappointing when teaching yoga doesn't feel as great as you expected when you're enrolled in your training.

Eventually it *does* feel incredible to teach a yoga class —to feel confident, happy, and authentic. Time stops and inspiration flows. It's one of my favorite feelings in the world. But honestly, I hardly ever felt that way during the first year —maybe two—of teaching. Instead, I often was nervous, insecure, preoccupied, and often with the lingering sensation that I hadn't quite nailed it. I was always relieved when class was over. It was only after a couple of hundred classes that I started to feel the great satisfaction of a well-taught class.

If you are struggling with any of the challenges I describe in this chapter, trust me that it gets much better, but never completely goes away. I still battle with these things, albeit much less often and much less intensely. Give it time and practice, and use these strategies to handle the new-teacher challenges with grace, wisdom, and ease.

Most of all, know that you are not alone. It's totally normal to feel less than calm during your first year of teaching. Struggling with these challenges is a sign of growth, not weakness.

Challenge: Feeling Like You Aren't a "Real" Yoga Teacher

Around the same time that I started teaching yoga, I enrolled in a workshop series on advanced *asana* taught by two awesome women, let's call them Katie and Lila. They knew a lot more than me about anatomy and sequencing, and they could do all these awesome poses that I could not. They were also very kind and friendly people, with flawless skin and very clear whites of their eyes, and I was totally intimidated by them. I felt like a geeky freshman and they were cool seniors. I felt self-conscious about calling myself a yoga teacher in comparison to them.

So I didn't. I didn't tell them that I was teaching classes, and I *really* did not want them to find out on their own. I imagined a scene where they would be like, "Jackie, *you*? Teach *yoga*?" looking baffled while a little mental blooper reel played of all times I failed at doing the advanced poses.

But keeping it secret proved to be tricky because I had already posted flyers for my class all around town, including at the shopping center where their studio was. Also, Lila had a day job and her office was located in the renovated mill building where I taught my yoga class. I knew it was only a matter of time.

Meanwhile at the workshop series, the longer I went without mentioning that I had recently completed my 200-hour training and was currently teaching classes, the more awkward I felt. This was especially true after the day they asked who else in class was a yoga teacher, and I didn't raise my hand. With every passing week, I walked quicker into the mill building to teach my classes, praying that I wouldn't bump into Lila leaving her office.

Inevitably, it happened. One winter evening, Lila was leaving her office as I was arriving. The jig was up. I was literally standing in front of a yoga studio with a flyer on the door that announced in 48-point font, "Yoga classes with Jackie Kinealy!" and in my hand, I was holding a stack of those same fliers. Cornered, I could feel the heat rising and my face turning red. The conversation went something like this:

"Hi Jackie!"
"HI! Oh my gosh, Lila?!"
"How are you? You teach in this studio, right? I've seen your flyers."
"Yep! Yeah, just one class a week. It's ok. Usually not many people come, hahahaha!"
"Oh well that's cool...." [Noticing my awkwardness]. Are you signing up for the next workshop series?"
"Yes! I am! I'm so excited about it!!"
"Ok, great. Well, I'll see you then."
"Ok cool! Bye!" [Turns and slams body into studio door, thinking it is unlocked]

Yeesh. Looking back, I can't believe how insecure I felt about calling myself a yoga teacher. Part of it, I think, was that I had such a poor teacher training that I felt unqualified. But there was a deeper layer to my insecurity. I felt like I wasn't the right type of person to be a yoga teacher. I felt not good enough—in my life and in my practice.

As you might expect then, feeling insecure wasn't limited to my interactions with Lila. In those early days, a little part of me always felt like an imposter while I was leading class. I worried I would say something incorrect, break a fundamental sequencing rule, or be unable to help a student modify a pose. I worried that I would be up there, talking away, while it slowly dawned on everyone that I wasn't a real yoga teacher.

Hindsight has shown me a few things. One, I'm much more secure as a person at 31 years old than I was at 25, thankfully. For me—and maybe for you too—a major part of overcoming insecurity was simply growing up. Two, feeling like an imposter motivated me to work my butt off—studying and practicing in order to earn a bit more credibility. Of course there is still an ocean of things I have yet to learn, but I can say I know much more than when I started.

Three, it is normal and healthy to feel like you don't know what you are doing *when you actually don't*! I was right to feel unsure of myself because there truly was a lot I didn't know. If you think you are doing a perfect job from the start, you aren't seeing yourself clearly. Basic teacher training can only prepare you so much. After that, the real information you need is hard-won and experience based. There are no shortcuts, only practice and time.

Overcome Feeling Like a Fraud: Work Like a Farmer

1. **Be honest about your weaknesses.** If you feel unprepared as a yoga teacher, you probably are, at least a bit. Pay attention to where there are gaps in your knowledge by writing down questions when they arise and looking up the answers.

2. **Remember what you do know.** At the same time, remember that you *do* know a good amount about yoga. At this point, you have probably been practicing for years and you

just completed a 200-hour training! You have some good stuff to share, and besides your most important role is providing space for people to practice. It's okay that you don't know everything.

3. **Study and practice.** Commit to studying or reading yoga books or articles for at least 20 minutes every day. Take as many classes as you can with all different sorts of teachers, and write down something you learn from each. The more inspiration you gather, the better a teacher you will be.

4. **Be humble.** If a student stumps you with a question, it's perfectly acceptable to say, "I don't know." In fact, it's the best response. Don't pretend to know more than you do. Tell them you will find out, and follow up next time. They won't think less of you, they will probably just be grateful that you care enough to find an answer.

5. **Trust the journey.** Know that those feelings of insecurity are a natural part of being new at something, and they will fade. It doesn't mean that something's wrong, or that you aren't cut out for this job. As you gain experience, you will feel more confident.

6. **Shift your focus.** Remember that people come to yoga for themselves, not to judge and criticize you. Concentrate on serving your students by teaching a good yoga class, not on what they are thinking about you, because they probably aren't.

Challenge: Getting Stage Fright

Jerry Seinfeld has a well-known joke that goes, "According to most studies, people's number one fear is public speaking. Number two is death. Death is number two. Does that sound right? This means to the average person, if you go to a funeral, you're better off in the casket than doing the eulogy!"

Public speaking is scary for a lot of people, and teaching yoga not only involves speaking in front of a group, but also demonstrating poses, setting the tone for class, and connecting with students. There is an element of performance in teaching yoga, and stage fright is a real challenge, even for those who have been doing it for a long time.

In school, I did all right with public speaking, but when I started teaching yoga it was different. I felt shy, and struggled to make eye contact with students. Subconsciously, I was worried that if I looked at their faces, I would read the message, "This class sucks." Also, I was too shy to speak about a theme—something I wanted to do because other teachers had inspired me with their class themes. I would prepare something to talk about before class, write it all out, and memorize it. Then when it came time to start class, I would bail and not talk about the theme at all, afraid of getting something wrong or sounding silly.

Today I mostly have overcome my stage fright, and you will too after you teach more classes and gain confidence. I still have days when I wish I could teach with a paper bag over my head—days when don't want anyone to look at me, when the right words won't come out of my mouth, when my voice sounds small and weak. In general, though, stage fright faded for me and it does for most people. If it never goes away completely, that's ok, too. A friend of mine has been teaching for 10 years, everyone loves him, and he still gets nervous before teaching a big class. However long it lasts, you can use these tips to ease your stage fright.

Overcome Stage Fright: Keep Calm and Carry On

1. **Breathe.** Before class, spend one or two minutes taking deep breaths with your feet firmly planted on the ground. Reign in your focus. Pray for guidance from your teachers, from God, and from your own inner wisdom.

2. **Speak to just one person.** If you're nervous about giving a talk or sharing a story, pretend you're speaking to just one specific person in your class—a friend or the person with whom you are most comfortable. Still do look around the room at the others, but pretend that you are talking to just that one friend.

3. **Make eye contact.** If you're shy about making eye contact, like I was (and sometimes still am), you just gotta do it. Make it a goal to look three people in the eye after you *namaste*. Force yourself to do it. You can also make it a habit to look around at people's faces when they are in a pose and focusing

more on their practice than on you.

4. **Talk to people outside of class.** I speak with more confidence during class if I have normal conversations with students before class. I also notice a correlation between how relaxed I feel teaching and how many people's names I know. When we joke around and tell each other about our lives, I feel like myself. Then during class, I feel more grounded, and my voice is clear and strong.

5. **Shift your focus.** Remind yourself that most people are thinking about themselves, not you, and they just want to do yoga. In the same vein, focus on your students instead of yourself. It's true that there are elements of performance to teaching—vocal quality, presence, charisma—but teaching is really a service you provide, not a performance you are making. Take the spotlight off yourself and shift your focus to teaching the best class you can for your students.

Challenge: Depending on Approval and Praise from Others

Sometimes I teach a class and think to myself, "Girl, you *nailed* that!" As people settle into *savasana*, I'm sitting there excited for everyone to tell me after class what a good job I just did. But then class ends, and everyone just packs up and leaves. Some people practically speed walk out of the studio while others give me a quick, "Thank you!" and a little wave.

Other times, I'll teach a class, and I'll think, "Oh dear God, that class was *horrible*." While people settle into *savasana*, I'm dreading interacting with them after class, embarrassed that I disappointed them. But then class ends, and people say, "That was such a great class! I feel so good!" or "Oh, that was just what I needed!"

It's confusing, and I am a people-pleaser, so the mismatched feedback can be disorienting. As such, my advice here is a reminder for myself, too: don't pay attention to the compliments or the snubs. They aren't a good measure of how good a job you did.

There are lots of reasons why students who had a great experience wouldn't stop to tell you about it. They are shy, they just want to go home, they're too relaxed, they don't think you need to hear it. On the flip side, some people will always say, "Great class," when it wasn't especially good. They say it to be polite, because they are uncomfortable with silence, they feel bad for you, or they sense that you need to hear it. You never know where compliments are coming from, so don't put too much stock in them.

Better to be your own judge of how you did, and learn to stand in your own approval. Did you try your best? Were you well prepared? Did you pay attention to your students? Did you try to give them what they needed? This is not to say that you should ignore all feedback. Certainly not. My advice is to focus on doing your best for your students and not try to get everyone to like you. It goes back to the distinction in Chapter 2 between teaching from a place of love instead of a place of fear. Tara Brach, the Buddhist meditation teacher describes in her book *Radical Acceptance* how this different mindset changes you:

> *When I remain aware that the Buddhist teachings are precious to me and that I love sharing them with others, I can throw myself into what I'm doing with enormous passion. But sometimes that voice of insecurity and unworthiness arises, and I listen to it. Suddenly writing or preparing a presentation is linked to winning or losing love or respect, and my entire experience of working shifts.....While I always intend to give a wholehearted effort, now that effort is wrapped in fear. I am anxiously striving to be good enough and to reap the rewards. My love for what I do becomes clouded over when working becomes a strategy to prove my worth.*

Overcome Depending on Praise: Learn To Stand in Your Own Approval

1. **Remember what you are doing.** Start each class by reading your mission statement, an inspirational quote, or a passage of a yoga book you love to refocus on what you want to give your students.

2. **Have your own definition of a "great class."** Create your own criteria you can use to tell yourself that you've done a good job. What does a "great class" look and feel like for you? One where you have done your best to prepare? One where you feel like you connect

with your students? One where you feel totally present and engaged? Define success for yourself and use that as your measure instead of depending on the ambiguous feedback.

3. **Don't take things personally.** Realize that a person's experience of what you teach has a lot to do with how they're feeling that day, their personality, their preferences, and how yoga "should" be. All you can do is offer the class with a clear intention, do your best, and then let go of how it lands with people.

Challenge: Thinking You Just Taught a Really Bad Class

Whether it's because I was tired of doing yoga that day, or feeling a little awkward for some reason, or because there was an unusual mix of students in the room, I have taught my share of "bad" yoga classes. Every now and then, people just don't seem into it, and I'm not excited about what we are doing either. It is inevitable.

But I have good news: a bad class is never as bad as you think. I have faith that most people just want to breathe, to move, to get some space, and to leave feeling better than when they walked in. They probably aren't aware of half of what you think you did badly. Plus (and I'm not sure if this is good news) I have noticed that if I am in a yoga class with a teacher I like, and I am not having a great practice, I usually assume it's because of *me* and how I am feeling, and not because the teacher is having an off-day. The point is that students are never going to be half as critical of you as you are of yourself.

Overcoming "Bad" Classes: Don't Take Yourself So Seriously

1. **Put it in perspective.** That was one single class out of many that you will teach. You probably won't even remember it in a week. Let it roll off your back.

2. **Learn from it.** Sit down for 5 or 10 minutes as soon as possible after the class and reflect. Why did you think it was wrong? Is it something you can work on improving, like your speaking voice? Or something you can avoid in the future, like not eating a big sandwich 30 minutes before class? Even if it's mostly in your head, there are things you can do to make it better next time.

3. **Realize that it's mostly in your head.** Sometimes if a student is lying in *savasana* with their eyes wide open staring at the ceiling, seemingly not relaxed or peaceful at all, I will think, "Oh my god, they hate me." But I know that's a ridiculous leap. Some people are simply more comfortable with their eyes open. Maybe something crazy is going on in their life. Whatever. Recognize when you are taking one thing, like a person's facial expression, and blowing it up into something else entirely.

Challenge: Getting Burnt Out

At one point, I was teaching yoga at a makeshift studio in a taekwondo school to which I biked twelve miles round trip three mornings a week. I had to set up and take down the decorations, candles, and lamps that made it feel like a yoga studio before and after class. Between the bike ride, the setup, teaching the class, talking to students afterward, and taking everything back down again, I worked practically all morning for $40. It was not sustainable.

There are lots of different ways to burn out. Maybe you are hungry for any opportunity, so you say yes to the class that's a 45-minute drive in rush hour, and you realize you just spent three hours for $25, minus taxes. Maybe you want to be a full-time instructor, so you end up teaching 17 classes a week at four different studios, which makes you exhausted and sick of yoga altogether. Maybe you want to teach as much as possible, but you can't quit your day job because you have a family, so you teach on evenings and weekends and you never have a break.

Avoiding burnout is tricky because when you are a new teacher, sometimes you have to cut your teeth by accepting the classes that other people don't want. Sometimes you have to say yes to the 6 a.m. classes, the small classes, the ones that don't pay well, the faraway studios. If you're holding out for perfect classes, you will never start working.

So what's the right balance? How can you work hard without burning out? I can't answer that for you. But I can offer questions to consider when deciding which classes to add to your schedule. You may realize that the commute is bad, the pay is not great, and the style is not your favorite, but you want it anyway. It's worth it to you. Or you may decide it's not the right fit. The criteria on the next page are to encourage you to be thoughtful before you commit.

Overcoming Burnout: Look Before You Leap

1. **Think it through.** Ask yourself the following questions before you commit to a class.

   - How does this class fit into my weekly schedule?
   - What will the commute be like? How long? Is it during rush hour?
   - Do I enjoy the studio, the students, and the style of yoga I would be teaching?
   - Can I see myself teaching this class weekly for at least a year?
   - What do other teachers say about working there?

2. **Take care of yourself.** Get sleep, eat well, and move your body every day. Don't burn the candle at both ends. Respect yourself.

3. **Conserve your energy.** Practice saying no to extra commitments that aren't important to you, when possible, to avoid wearing yourself too thin.

Challenge: Losing Your Inspiration

Every few weeks, I get into a funk where I feel like I teach the same poses all the time, repeat the same cues, and organize class according to the same structure. When that happens, I don't feel excited to teach, and I'm anxious that my students are bored and annoyed, even though as a student I often enjoy doing familiar things in my favorite classes.

There is a difference between keeping some of the same effective elements in each class because they work well and teaching the same stuff every week because you don't have any new ideas. Students can tell when you're not into it. When you're bored by what you're teaching, there's no magic in your class for anyone else.

For me, there's a direct connection between losing my inspiration as a teacher and being stalled as a student—skipping my morning home practice, not going to other people's classes, and not making an effort to learn something new every day. Luckily, there are easy solutions to the problem of losing your inspiration.

Overcome Losing Inspiration: Explore and Learn

1. **Read every damn day.** Commit to reading one section of a book or a yoga article every day. I always find something good at Yoga International online. I also go through phases when I read at least ten pages of a book on spirituality or philosophy every morning.

2. **Take other people's classes.** Attend at least three classes each week with your favorite teachers, or practice with videos online.

3. **Expand your horizons.** Study a variety of movements like other types of yoga, Qi Gong, and different forms of dance. You'll be inspired by new ways of moving, and you can incorporate them into your classes.

4. **Don't reinvent the wheel.** You don't have to make everything 100 percent new each class. You use a template, keep some foundational movements, and also weave in new things. Creative cues, sequences, and pose variations, mixed with classics is a great formula.

Challenge: Having an Existential Crisis

I was the news editor of the student newspaper in college. I poured myself into the job, and I imaged that I wanted to be a reporter after graduation. The summer before graduation, I had an internship at a small newspaper in rural Missouri. One week, I spent hours writing an article about state budget cuts and the effect on the school district. The piece ran on the front page, and I was proud of it.

Later that night, though, I sat alone in my apartment feeling deflated. Most people probably only read the first couple of paragraphs of the story, if that much. Some read the whole thing, but either way, it wasn't going to change anything. The budget cuts were already set, and

the legislature wasn't going to reconsider anything because of an article by a college intern at a
small-town paper.

From there, I spiraled downward toward existential crisis. Even if I worked hard enough to
become a reporter for *The New York Times*, would
those stories make a difference? Reporters write
stories every day highlighting injustice, but the
world is still unjust. As my existential crisis un-
raveled, I wrote a rambling and angsty journal
entry, the gist of which was: what's the point?

Still, I completed the internship, writing
hard-hitting pieces about a dog biting a woman's
hand and description of a helicopter ride I took.
When summer ended, I returned to school to
finish my degree. I went back to working in the
newspaper office, staying there until 1 a.m. most
nights and waking up in the mornings in a near
panic about that evening's deadlines. The de-
mands of daily life covered up the din of my existential crisis, but when it came time to apply for
jobs, I couldn't do it.

I see in hindsight that reporters, of course,
make a huge difference for society. We absolutely
need journalists, and I am grateful to the men
and women who do a stressful job because they
are dedicated to the truth and to holding people
in power accountable. It's just not the job for me.
I like to feel like I'm directly helping people, and
I think that's true for most yoga teachers.

To generalize further, yoga teachers are
thoughtful people who gravitate toward this job
because they want to feel purposeful in their
work. We want to feel like what we do helps the
world. To put it another way, no one ever became

a yoga teacher for the money. And if they did, they were quickly disappointed.

That is why it can be so disheartening when you are a new teacher, and the job is not what you imagined at first.

For one, it takes a while to be good at it. Secondly, sometimes you end up working in settings that make you feel like a fitness instructor. Not that there's anything wrong with that, but you probably signed up for a more holistic role. Three, students don't always give you feedback even if they had an amazing experience, so it's difficult to tell if you are making an impact at all. Finally, if you teach a ton of classes and get over-stressed, you can lose touch with the big picture.

Here are some ways that I have found to pull myself out of existential spirals.

Overcoming Existential Dilemmas: Pay Attention and Stay Connected

1. **Read your mission statement.** Read your mission statement. Stay focused on the true purpose of teaching yoga and why it's important to you.

2. **Keep up your practice.** There is no quicker way to lose your inspiration for teaching yoga than to let your own practice lapse. Keep going to class with other teachers, practice with videos, practice at home on your own.

3. **Chart your progress.** After each class you teach, write down one thing you learned in a journal or notebook—something that worked,

something that didn't, something to try next time. Seeing yourself improve is motivating.

4. **Be discerning about jobs.** Looks for places aligned with your values, personality, and goals. Here you will thrive and stay inspired.

5. **Be patient.** Put in the hard work, keep your intentions clear, and trust that over time you will grow into the teacher you want to be.

6. **Remember, yoga is good!** Yoga really does help people feel better. Even the "bad" yoga classes I have attended have been fairly pleasant. I still got to move and breathe and have some space away from the grind.

Kind Vibes

Do you know someone who is so calm and grounded that simply being around them makes you feel calm and grounded too? As an instructor, if you come to class relaxed and present your students will feel at ease and receptive as well. If you are nervous, anxious, or preoccupied with how you're coming off, they will pick up on that.

Yoga students notice the quality of your energy and the tone of your voice more than your expertly crafted sequences. Not to say that intelligent sequencing and thoughtful instruction don't matter; they do. But don't get so caught up in nailing the performance of a perfect sequence that you forget that you are teaching real people.

Especially when you're brand new, it can be easy to lose touch with the service-based core of what you are doing amidst all the other stuff—finding jobs, making a good impression, figuring out how to make a living, commuting to the studio, planning classes, choosing music, establishing your teaching style. When yourself losing touch, pause, and remember that people in yoga class just want to breathe and move their bodies in a thoughtful way. They want a teacher who is authentic and present, so when you feel nervous, take a few deep breaths and try just to be yourself. Refer back to Chapter 2 for a refresher on the importance of service.

You Can Do It!

In this chapter, I have shared specific strategies and habits to overcome the myriad challenges of being a new yoga teacher, but in general, it's about three things: courage, focused effort, and patience. You have to get up every morning and commit to doing the best you can today, despite everything else that's going on. You have to plan and teach each class like it's the only one, while at the same time understanding that you teach many, many classes before you master the art of teaching yoga. It is your mindset that makes the difference.

Courage

Having courage means you are brave enough to be vulnerable—to get out there and do something you love even though you are scared to do it. It is *scary* to get in front of a room full of people and do anything, much less teach an hour-long yoga class. Having courage means teaching from your heart, even if you worry about people judging you. It means not letting your fear of how others receive what you give stop you from giving it.

If it makes you feel better, most people are just happy to be told what to do in a quiet room. They didn't show up to class to critique you, they just want to do yoga, and they probably won't notice the things you think you screwed up.

Still, you can't please everyone, and some people simply won't like your style of teaching. You can't take it personally because it's not really about you. Different people just have different preferences. It's unavoidable, no matter how good a teacher you become. For example, a couple of years ago I went to a workshop led by a popular, famous yoga teacher, and I just didn't like it. Undeniably, he is a master of yoga, but I didn't connect with his personality or teaching style. I didn't like the pace of his class or his vibe. But plenty of people at the workshop love him. So even the best teachers have people who don't like their class—just part of the gig.

Focused Effort

Focused effort means working hard on what matters. It is so easy to get stuck in "the thick of thin things," as Stephen Covey put it, where you are very busy all the time, but not doing the things that really matter. You get caught up in promoting yourself on social media, using valuable time you could have spent planning your classes. Or you find yourself preoccupied with a particular student who seemed not to like your class instead of evaluating how *you* think it went.

To practice focused effort, first you need to define your purpose and your values as we did with the mission statement earlier. Once you have a clear intention and good priorities, remind yourself what they are at the start of each week when you are preparing for your classes. Remind yourself frequently what you are hoping to provide for people—what your job is. The habit will help you stay in the healthy and life-affirming zone of service and other-centeredness, and out of the icky and crazy-making zone of ego and self-promotion.

Then, do your best to prepare for your classes so that they reflect your intention, priorities, and commitment to service. After each class, reflect on what went well and what you could improve. Stay tuned—in the next chapter, we explore staying on track with tools to improve. Yay!

Patience

Being patient means keeping it up for years! Years! There's no shortcut to becoming a great teacher who consistently delivers awesome classes, who is authentic and comfortable in her role, who is skillful and adaptable. The way forward is just time and lots of practice. You have to teach, teach, teach, teach and teach some more. You have to read books, learn from your mistakes, go to lots of classes, do continuing education, practice your cueing, hone your pacing, and more.

The thing is, there's no finish line; there is always more to learn. So enjoy the process and the thrill of seeing yourself improve, slowly but surely, your whole life long.

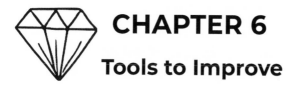

CHAPTER 6
Tools to Improve

"Do the best you can until you know better.
Then when you know better, do better."

-Maya Angelou

I bike most places I go, and what I love about biking versus driving is that it reminds me of the miraculous difference between living things and machines. Every day that I ride my bike, I get a little faster. My living tissues—my leg muscles, my heart, my lungs—rebound from the stress of the bike ride and grow stronger. Not so with machines. Every time I drive the car, I wear it down a little and decrease the life of the engine. Unlike my body, the car doesn't get stronger and better the more I drive it.

The process of growth is amazing. When you do something physically challenging, like biking up a hill or lifting heavy weights or running a far distance, the effort actually damages your muscle fibers and makes your body sore. But then you rest, your tissues bounce back stronger and healthier than they were before! How incredible that life works that way, that living things fight to thrive.

The same process exists for growing and improving as a yoga teacher. When you first start teacher training, learning a skill as basic as cueing people into a pose is really hard. Just this past weekend, I watched a group of 200-hour trainees play a yoga charades game where they took turns picking scraps of paper with pose names on them from a bowl and guiding everyone into the pose using no demonstration, no pose names, and no filler-language. They really struggled with it. People flushed red, froze, and totally blanked. But in a year, I'm sure most of them will look back and be amazed that it was so hard.

What you practice you improve. You already know this, you just need to remind yourself of it when your inner "gremlins" try to tell you that you are naturally bad at teaching yoga. You are not—you just need more practice. You can adopt specific habits and practices to improve your skills, just like an athlete does drills, and feel yourself improving every day from the practice. Put in the hard work. Rest. Reflect on what you learned. Do it better the next time.

Some of the following practices you will want to practice daily, some weekly, some monthly. Regardless, be consistent and keep specific goals in mind to provide yourself the structure you need to really focus your efforts and make the improvements you want.

Record Yourself Teaching, Then Take Your Own Class

This one is super helpful, albeit a little painful. Once a month, bring a small voice recorder or your phone into class with you and record yourself teaching. If possible, and not too intrusive, video yourself teaching. Later at home, listen to or view the recording and take the class you just taught. Notice your cadence, your language, your volume, and the clarity of your instruction. Take notes. Sometimes it takes listening to your own voice to notice that you are off tempo, or holding the pose on the first side longer than the second.

If you have ever cringed listening to the sound of your own voice leaving a message, this might not be your favorite activity, but I believe it's one of the most helpful things you can do to improve your instruction. If you can do it once per month, you will learn so much about how you can improve your teaching.

Take Notes After Every Class

If you write down something you learned after every class you *take* and every class you *teach,* you will build an incredibly valuable resource for yourself. I am not always disciplined enough to take notes after every single class, but I do for most classes. Sometimes I write a theme or phrase like, "Effort is necessary, straining is not." Sometimes I record a particular sequence that I liked. Other times I write a couple of paragraphs on what made a class particularly robust or dull. When I'm planning the next week's classes, I can look back at my notes for ideas.

Start a notebook specifically for collecting lessons, inspirations, and insights. Try it for one month—write down a little bit about each class you teach or take. Steal a beautiful cue from another teacher, congratulate yourself for remembering students' names, remind yourself not to ever start a class *that* way again. Each entry can be three words or a whole page. Do it, and you will cultivate a mindset of continuous learning and growth. You will track your progress, solidify your teaching style and philosophy, and collect beautiful little gems—great pose combinations, unexpected transitions, inspiring music, interesting cues, feel-good assists—that are easy to forget unless you write them down.

Seek Honest Feedback

An honest friend is an asset; they tell you what you need to hear. My best friend from college Clare is brutally honest with me, especially when it comes to my thrift-store clothing purchases. One evening, she was sitting on my bed drinking cheap wine while I raked through my closet choosing an outfit for the night. I pulled out a faux-velvet jumpsuit circa 1972 that was hot pink on top with a flower pattern like couch upholstery. It also featured a drawstring neckline (yes, neckline) and an empire waist.

Bafflingly as it seems to me now, on that particular night I couldn't decide whether it was the right outfit to impress a boy I liked. I held it up and turned toward Clare, who looked me right in the eye. "Jackie Kinealy," she said. "You should definitely not wear that jumpsuit."

Indeed, I should definitely not have worn that jumpsuit, and I did not wear that jumpsuit, thanks to Clare. We all need a friend who will tell us not to wear the jumpsuit. It's great to have a few friends who can give you honest feedback, including when it comes to teaching yoga. Find a feedback partner—preferably another yoga teacher who will come to your classes and be genuine enough to celebrate what you did well while pointing out what you can improve. Asking a more experienced teacher to come to your class and give you a review is also very helpful.

The feedback can be informal, or you can create a rubric, which is helpful if you are shy about critiquing each other. A rubric provides criteria and permission to talk about specific elements of the class. Below are ideas for rubric categories.

Voice quality. Could you hear me? Was my voice strong enough? Too loud? Too soft? Did I modulate my voice as appropriate for the sections of the class?

Language. Were my cues easy to understand? Any that were particularly helpful? Were any parts of class confusing? Did I speak succinctly? Did I use filler words, like *now we're gonna, from here, when you're ready, ums,* and *-ings*?

Sequence. Was the class appropriate for the level and style? Did the class flow smoothly from one section to another? Did any place feel rushed, awkward, or too slow? Did you sense a peak in energy to the class?

Balance. Was there a good mix of soothing and challenging poses? Did the class feel complete?

Connection. Did you feel welcome in the class? Did I smile, make eye contact, greet students? Did I make myself available after class?

Presence. Did I hold space well? Walk around the room? Set a good tone? Overall, how was my presence?

Collaborate

Another great, free way to develop your teaching skills is to organize informal workshops with your peers where you work on things like giving hands-on adjustments, instructing new poses, teaching class with no demonstration, and instructing poses when everyone has their eyes closed so can see where your verbal cues could be more clear.

You will save hundreds of dollars for continuing education courses this way, and you create an environment of collaboration and support among your fellow yoga teachers rather than one of competition.

Find a Mentor

Your mentor doesn't have to be your *guru*, and the relationship doesn't have to be formal.

You don't have to be the Karate Kid and Mr. Miyagi. A mentor simply can be a more experienced yoga teacher with whom you have chemistry, and whose teaching style you enjoy. Go to their classes regularly and build a friendship. Eventually, you could approach them for advice, or ask for coffee. As your relationship deepens, you might ask them to be your official mentor, but you don't have it. Formal mentorship can put a lot of pressure on the person, so if you have a good thing going without putting a label on it, you might just want to let it be.

Look It Up When
You Don't Know

My brother is in medical school, and last time he was home I noticed that he had this quote taped on the top rim of his laptop: "If you aren't sure how two steps are causally connected, you've uncovered a gap in your knowledge." In other words, when you see that two things are related but you don't know why, you have stumbled on a learning opportunity.

Whenever you find yourself asking "Why?" you are in a golden zone. Write down your question and look up the answer. Why do some Yin students struggle so much in Saddle pose, and others are totally fine? Which poses are best for low back pain? Should you really not do a headstand on your period? This is an amazing way to expand your knowledge.

Go to New and Different Classes

A few months ago I had coffee with a student who was considering enrolling in teacher training and she had a few questions about it before she signed up. She asked me if being a yoga teacher had ruined the experience of simply taking a yoga class—getting totally out of my head—or if I was constantly thinking about how the teacher was teaching the class.

The answer is yes and no. Yes, when I take a class there is usually a little ticker tape running along the bottom of my mind, like on CNN. *Good cue! Remember to write that down. This music is a little too loud. I wonder what the pose is a prep for. Ah, I like this pose sequence!* Before teacher training, I didn't have that ticker tape. But also, no. No, it doesn't necessarily ruin the experience of taking a class. It still feels great to take a great class.

Go to classes with new and different yoga teachers because there is something to learn from each one. Last week I went to a new class at a heated studio. I don't normally practice hot or power yoga, so it kicked my butt, mostly in a good way. Afterward, the teacher gave me a high-five. I loved that! I don't think I have ever high-fived a student, but now I might start.

Going to lots of classes as a student can also help you take some pressure off yourself by reminding you that yoga usually feels pretty damn good, even if the teacher isn't amazing and the class is only average. When I don't make time to go to a few classes a week, I forget about this fact. But then I go to a class and I realize that yoga doesn't need to be dressed up. It's good just plain.

It's like an heirloom tomato at the peak of tomato season. Sure, it's delicious with salt, pepper, and olive oil. It makes an amazing sauce. Pizza, yes! But it's also great by itself.

Read One Yoga Book a Month

Good yoga books are rocket fuel. In your classes, it's good to mix in a few new cues and pose variations each week, and if you stay well-stocked with yoga books, it will be much easier to keep your teaching fresh. Consistently reading, even a few pages a week, has given me tons of bright ideas, especially when I'm in a rut.

The important part is making it a habit. Every week try to schedule 30 minutes to an hour of reading and note-taking. You could also read 10 pages of a book every morning or every evening, which will put you on track to read one yoga book per month.

Practice Teaching with a Metronome

I know, I am full of fun ideas. Google free online metronome, select the right tempo, and practice teaching along to the beat. This is particularly helpful for Vinyasa teachers. A terrific flow class has a steady, even cadence throughout. You are the drummer and your students are the ensemble. The steady pace feels effortless to the students, but it takes practice and focus to maintain for the teacher. If you add a cue or your mind wanders for a moment, the breath becomes lopsided and you lose momentum. Practicing with a metronome helps you build strong internal timing and tempo.

Mentally Repeat Each Student's Name in *Savasana*

When your students are in *savasana*, what do you do? Sometimes I like to sit quietly and look around the room at each person, mentally saying their name and wishing them well. There are two benefits to this practice. First, you cultivate loving-kindness toward your students, which I believe they can feel. Second, it's a good way to memorize people's names, which is important if you want to connect in a real way. Besides you have to do *something* sitting there, right?

Ask Your Students Questions

At the moment, one of my favorite things to teach is a two-hour workshop called Yoga 101 which is geared toward people who are new to yoga and want a thorough, friendly, no-pressure introduction to the basic poses, class format, and studio etiquette. I start the workshop by going around the room, having everyone say their name, what they are hoping to learn today, and what they want from a yoga practice in general. During the class, I pause to see if there are any questions, and I encourage students to stop me if something is unclear.

I love getting to hear what people want from yoga, what is difficult for them, and what is confusing. Since I have been practicing yoga for a while, I sometimes forget what is hard at first. As a teacher, I sometimes get wrapped up in planning a sophisticated sequence or nerding out with the cues, and I forget that people really just want to move, stretch, get some stress relief, and find some peace.

Make a habit of asking your students questions about their practices. Especially when you have a new student, take a couple of minutes to ask them why they decided to try yoga. Why now? Also talk to longtime students about why they continue practicing. The more you understand what draws other people to yoga and what keeps them coming back, the better of a teacher you will be.

Use Positive Visualization

If you are nervous about teaching, spend a few minutes every day visualizing yourself teaching an amazing classes. Sit down, close your eyes, and picture yourself walking to the front of the room to start class—confident, relaxed, and warm. Picture yourself connecting with each student with eye contact and a smile. Imagine the whole class becoming absorbed in your instruction. Physically *feel* what it's like to be in a really great yoga class, where everything is flowing and time stands still. Then tell yourself, "You can do this. This is going to happen." And then go make it happen!

Take Care of Yourself

My good friend Lizzie is also a yoga teacher, and one week she was subbing a lot of classes. Lizzie is great at going slow, listening to her body, and resting when she needs it instead of pushing harder. I asked her how her week was going and she said, "It's doable if I practice exquisite self-care." That phrase stuck with me, and now I am stealing it for my book.

Practicing great self-care is important for all of us, and perhaps yoga teachers especially. Fill your cup so you have the capacity to give to others. Taking time to "slow down, enjoy life, and be well," as Shel Pink writes in her book *Slow Beauty*. Self-care is vital to your role as a yoga teacher because it is a physically and mentally demanding job. You need time to rest and recover. But self-care plays an even more central role. How *well* you feel—in your body and your soul—is essential to effective yoga teaching. You are a role model, in your words and actions, and also in the more subtle way that your energy comes across, and how you take care of yourself matters.

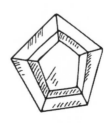

You Can Do It!

You will be amazed at how much you grow during your first year of teaching yoga. Honestly, you would improve a lot over the course of a year even if you didn't use any of the tools in this chapter, and just taught three yoga classes every week. But you will improve exponentially if you are strategic and thoughtful about ways that you can channel your energy and focus.

Of course, you don't have to use all of these tools. Pick the two or three that sound the most exciting and try them out for a month. Then you can decide to keep it up or swap them out. You also might find other practices not listed here that are helpful for you. The important thing is staying in a mindset of growth; remember how far you have come and have faith in how far you can go.

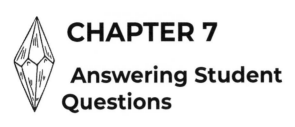

CHAPTER 7

Answering Student Questions

"So many of us believe in perfection which ruins everything else because the perfect is not only the enemy of the good, it's also the enemy of the realistic, the possible and the fun."

-Rebecca Solnit

Right now, you probably don't *feel* like an expert. Regardless, many students will *think* you are one. After all, you are standing in the role of a yoga teacher, and you are the person folks will come to with questions. Inevitably, people will ask you questions that you don't know how to answer. Not knowing is stressful, but also completely normal.

During my first year of teaching, I would get nervous when students came up after class to ask me questions. I worried that I wouldn't know the answer and would be exposed as a fraud. One time, a couple of minutes before class started, a woman told me she had a bruised coccyx and wanted to know how she could modify around it. I had no idea. I had never even heard of someone bruising their coccyx. I don't remember what I said, but it was probably something like,

"Um, sit on a blanket!" And then I probably walked away.

Some other questions that stumped me during my first year teaching include:

- Is it okay if my kneecap faces off center during Half Moon Pose?
- Why does my low back hurt when I do low lunge?
- Is it okay for my hands to face outward in Downward Dog?
- Can you show me some modifications for my arthritis?
- I thought yoga would help my shoulder pain. Why is it making it worse?
- Am I doing this right?

Fresh out of teacher training, I was not prepared to answer these questions—at least not on the spot. Sometimes I did have the answer somewhere in my head, but I felt frozen and slightly panicky in the moment, and I couldn't access that information. Other times, I truly had no idea.

I thought a *real* yoga teacher would be able to answer any question about any person's body in any pose, all the time. That I couldn't made me feel like a total rookie, which I absolutely was.

The real rookie mistake was believing in the first place that I should know the exact right answer to every question. Experienced teachers know that's impossible. Answering student questions doesn't work that way. People's bodies are varied and complex, and you shouldn't expect to know why, for example, the arch of someone's foot hurts in Warrior I—at least not without more information.

I repeat: you almost always need more information to supply a helpful answer. When a student asks you a question, that's the starting point of a conversation, not your cue to spit back an anatomy book answer. The anatomy book answer usually is not very helpful anyway. Instead, you should respond to student questions with some questions of your own. If you remember one thing from this chapter, let it be this: **ask questions before you give answer.**

Asking questions gives you as the instructor a better understanding of what's really going on and gives your student the opportunity to cultivate better body awareness. Then the two of you together can discover a solution.

Asking questions also means you don't have to study and cram, or prepare answers to the thousands of possible questions that students might lob at you. Instead, you can take a general approach. Imagine three big buckets or types of questions that people ask:

1. Why does this hurt?

2. Why can't I do this?

3. Am I doing this right?

Once you understand which type of question your student is asking, you can understand the type of conversation you need to have. Focus on starting conversations and forging connections instead of establishing your expertise or being right.

Category One: Why Does This Hurt?

The Question

Chapter 8 will focus on modifying for various common injuries. In this chapter, let's focus on what to do when a student asks you why something hurts. I have been stumped many times by students telling me about various body parts that hurt: wrists, shoulders, foot arch, neck. Just this week, one of my regular students told me that his left elbow joint felt like it needed to pop but can't in Downward Dog. I honestly had no idea what to tell him.

Determining the cause of someone's pain can be complex, individualized, and above your paygrade. So what should you do when a student asks why something hurts?

The Answer

First, you need more information—you need to ask questions. An ache that initially seems mysterious might make sense after you learn, for example, that the person had knee surgery five years ago and forgot to mention it to you. Asking questions also encourages the student to be more aware of the sensation by requiring them to describe the specific location and what it feels like. Here are some questions to get started.

💎 Did the pain start recently, or have you always had it in this pose?

💎 Point to where it hurts.

💎 Does it feel like the pain is in your muscles or near the joint?

💎 Is the pain sharp or dull?

💎 Does it feel tingly? Pinching? Achy?

💎 Have you had an injury or surgery there before?

💎 What happens to the pain when you move around and adjust the pose a little?

Second, ask the person to demonstrate the pose for you and experiment with modifications. A really common complaint is wrist pain in Downward Dog. If a student asks you about this, have her do the pose. If you see that she's dumping weight into her upper body and jamming the heel of her palm into the ground, point it out. Then instruct how to use the abdominal muscles to lift weight out of the shoulders and wrists, and to seal more of her palm to the mat.

If that doesn't work, ask her to try variations—bending the knees, adjusting the hands and feet. Grab a set of blocks. Try a bunch of stuff and go slow. Make it a conversation by offering suggestions and having the student describe how the sensation changes as you go. Hopefully, the two of you will be able to find something that feels better for her wrists. Then the next time she does Downward Dog, she is equipped with functional, first-hand information on what helps her wrist pain—much more than if you had rattled off something about pressing into her knuckle mounds and left it there.

Side note: if your student describes the pain as sharp and dangerous-feeling, they shouldn't do the pose. Give a different option that doesn't hurt, and recommend they get it checked out by a professional.

After you have asked questions and explored variations and none of it helped, it's okay to say that you don't know how to fix it, and help direct them to someone who can. The cause of someone's pain is often complex, and sometimes beyond your expertise as a new instructor. With my student's elbow-popping, I Googled it and found a forum of physical therapists discussing similar cases, and they were also stumped. That made me feel better about being unable to answer his question. You do your students a service when you acknowledging that something is above your level of expertise.

Category Two: Why Can't I Do This?

The Question

Social media gets blamed for everything, but it really *is* to blame for making it seem like if you practice enough yoga, you can do any crazy pose, and that the crazy poses are important in and of themselves. Models and former gymnasts with exceptional, uncommon flexibility and joint mobility post photos of themselves doing insane backbends or splits or arm balances, and the regular people who see them want to look like that.

My friend recently started teaching private lessons to a woman who had never practiced yoga. On their first meeting showed her a picture of a yoga model in Scorpion Pose—the forearm balance where your legs are bent and staggered—and asked, "How soon can we get me to this?"

Not that working toward a challenging pose is bad. It builds discipline, and it can be rewarding and fun. What *is* bad—or at least misguided—is the belief that everybody can do every yoga pose if they are devoted enough, which simply is not true. Some people are able to put their feet behind their heads not because they are better yogis (or better people for that matter) but because of the way their pelvis and femur bones are shaped. No amount of practice or intention-setting can compensate for that. In the same way, the depth of your backbends can have *much* more to do with the distance between your vertebrae than your devotion to your practice.

The point is that every person's body is unique. Therefore, everyone's yoga practice is unique. In the past few decades, the western yoga world has ignored the reality of human variation by focusing too much on standardized alignment cues that don't work for everybody. Bernie Clark explains this trend really well in his book *Your Body, Your Yoga*. This same mindset leads students and teachers alike to falsely believe that every person is capable of doing any pose, if only they practice enough.

Of course, it is also true that practice does make people more flexible, stronger, and able to do poses that they couldn't do when they started yoga. If people didn't make progress and improve, it wouldn't be very rewarding. The trick is being able to tell the difference when your students ask, "Why?"

The Answer

Usually, the students who ask, "Why can't I do that?" have been coming to class for a while, and they are seeing themselves improve in other parts of their practice. They feel stronger, more flexible, and successful in most poses, and they get frustrated when they can't do something. They want to know why, and how to fix it.

When someone asks you why they can't do something, as the instructor it's your job to ask why back.

1. Why they are asking in the first place?
2. What's going on in their body?
3. Why does it matter?

First, why they are asking? One time, a regular Yin student asked me why she could barely fold forward at all in Dragonfly pose, the Yin version of Wide-Angle Seated Forward Bend. She barely tipped forward from her hips while most other people had their forearms on the ground. I asked her where she felt the stretch, if anywhere, in the pose. She said her inner thighs felt stretched. That's one of the main target areas of the pose, so to me, there's not a problem. But we talked a little longer and it became clear that she was asking because she didn't like the fact that she couldn't fold forward like everyone else. I encouraged her to focus on the function of the pose, the stretch, rather than how she thought the pose should look.

That brings us to the second why: why is this happening anatomically? In the Dragonfly example, the answer, at least partially, hinges on figuring out whether the resistance the person is feeling is due to tension in the tissues or compression at the bones, another principle from Paul Grilley and Bernie Clark.

Both tension and compression limit mobility, but tension can be overcome and compression cannot. Tension is felt in the tissues, and often in the direction opposite from the movement. For example, when you do a forward fold, you feel the stretch in the back of your body. When you do a backbend, you feel the stretch in the front of the body. Tension in the fascia and the muscles can be changed over time with consistent practice. If a runner with tight hamstrings starts coming regularly to a yoga class, he will likely be able to fold deeper as the weeks go on and he stretches his tight tissues.

Compression, on the other hand, limits mobility because one part of the body is coming into contact with another part of the body. For example, if a flexible student does a forward fold and her chest is touching her thighs, she can't go any farther, period. There is a fundamental and obvious block. Think of the same principle in the joints when bone reaches compression with bone. When the head of the femur bone rotates in the hip socket, it reaches compression with the socket at different points with different individuals, a fact that cannot be changed with any amount of practice. It's how the bones are structured. Everyone's skeleton is different, so everyone reaches compression at different places.

In *Your Body, Your Yoga*, Clark writes that you can't know simply by looking at your students whether someone is experiencing tension or compression because you don't have X-ray vision. You can, however, help your students learn how to pay attention to their own bodies and determine the answer for themselves, a concept Clark calls WSM, "What's Stopping Me." He says that the best gift you can give your students is the skill to determine for themselves what's going on in their body.

Next time this comes up, ask your student to carefully come into the pose and describe the sensation they are feeling. If tension is to blame, Clark writes, it will usually be quite obvious to the student, felt in the belly of the muscles or at the tendon closer to the bone. To overgeneralize, it will feel like a stretch. If compression is the culprit, the sensation might be more difficult to pinpoint and describe. It might feel like pinching, stuck, hard, and very localized.

Going back to the Dragonfly example, I asked my Yin student to do a few other stretches— Bound Angle, Seated Forward Fold, a side bend— and based on her flexibility in other shapes and how she described the sensation, I guessed that the reason she couldn't fold deeper was due to compression at the hip joint. I propped her pelvis up higher with a bolster, which gave her a little more depth in the fold, but I think that the real solution was helping her understand that there wasn't truly a problem, and to focus on how the pose feels rather than how it looks.

Now we arrive at third why: why it matters. Sometimes all you have to do is to remind students that achieving the pose isn't the point. Regardless of what's stopping them—tension or compression—how the pose looks often isn't important. Focus instead on how the pose feels. Are they feeling the intended effect? If so, then leave it be. If not, what modification or alternate pose will achieve that intended effect? If a student wants to do a party trick pose, that's cool. You can help them figure out how to work toward it. But temper it with reminders that achieving the poses alone isn't the point, and remember that your job is to focus on function rather than aesthetic.

Category Three: Am I Doing This Right?

The Question

Sometimes students (especially new students) preoccupy themselves with doing a pose "right." I don't mean when someone feels discomfort or pain in a pose and thinks, "This can't be it," and I'm not talking about when people are confused about what the teacher is asking them to do.

I'm talking when students are so worried about how the pose *looks*, and exactly right, that they ignore how the pose *feels*. I am talking about the difference between doing the pose from the outside-in versus the inside-out.

In the early days of my yoga practice, I was in class at a gym where the yoga studio had a wall of mirrors. At the time, I was just starting to get really passionate about yoga, and I was feeling great in Warrior II—strong, open and relaxed. My normal studio didn't have mirrors, so when I glanced at myself in the mirror that day I was surprised to see my rear sticking way out. I had been practicing just long enough to know that I should "tuck my tailbone," and I thought that I had been! I looked at myself in the mirror and tried to make the pose look right, but I just couldn't do it. I could tuck, but then my bent knee swayed inward. I could move my knee wider, but then I came untucked. I couldn't do both at the same time.

"Am I doing this right?" I asked the teacher after class, "Why can't I tuck my tailbone? It feels like it pulls my knee out of alignment when I do." In hindsight, she must have been fairly to teaching new because she got this stricken look on her face, a look that I recognize now as the panic of a recent YTT graduate trying to keep it together.

Without missing a beat, she spit out the standard instructions for Warrior II, demonstrated quickly and then literally just walked away. I am laughing writing this because I know that I *absolutely* pulled a similar move when I was brand new. But *you,* my friend, can do better.

The Answer

What would have been a better way for the instructor to answer my question? Alignment-based teachers may disagree, but I believe that a good answer to the question "Am I doing this right?" is, "That depends. How does it feel?"

When I asked about my Warrior II, the teacher at the gym could have responded with something like, "Well, how does the pose feel to you?" and then asked me to show her. She could have asked me to level my pelvis, engage my core, take my knee toward my baby toe to see what happened to my hips. Then she could have asked about pain in my lower back, knees, and hip joints. If I had none, she could have told me that my pose is fine how it is, even if it doesn't look perfect—because there's no such thing as a perfect pose. If we had a few extra minutes, she could have had me demonstrate a pose where my femur bones were in a similar position, externally rotated and abducted, like Frog pose, to check my flexibility there.

I later learned that a possible explanation for why I can't get my tailbone directly under my body in Warrior II could be compression—the way my femur bone fits into my hip socket, which no amount of stretching or adjusting can change. When I flex and abduct my hip, as in Warrior II, my femur bone hits up against the outer rim of its socket, and I can't move it any farther. That bone-on-bone compression makes it hard to keep my legs in Warrior II while simultaneously lengthening my tailbone.

Now, I am not saying that my 24-Hour Fitness teacher should have spent 20 minutes running tests to figure out how the head of my femur bone fits into my hip socket. I'm saying she could have helped me notice how the pose feels in my own body while reminding me of its intended effects, and making sure it wasn't painful.

The moral of the story is don't just say yes or no when someone asks you if they are doing something right, especially if you aren't sure. You don't have to be an expert on every person's body in every pose. In fact, you can't be! Instead take a few minutes to look at the pose, explore variations, see how their body moves, and ask how it feels. Do that, and you will both learn something.

You Can Do It!

I used to dread students asking questions, afraid that I wouldn't know the answer and I would expose myself as an imposter who didn't know anything about anything. I expected a *real* teacher to be able to immediately answer any question from any student at any time, which was misguided because there usually isn't a single answer to a question, especially regarding someone else's body. So take the pressure off yourself! Talk to your students as people. Start a conversation and find a solution together. If you still don't know, it's OK to say, "I don't know, but I'll find out."

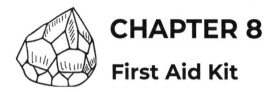

CHAPTER 8

First Aid Kit

"The only way to glean knowledge is contemplation, and the road to that is time. There's nothing else. It's just time."

-Maria Papova

When I first started teaching, I would ask students before class if they had injuries. It didn't hurt to ask, I suppose, but it also didn't help much because I usually didn't know what to do with the answer. One time, a woman told me that she had arthritis in her knees that made it very painful to bend them. I nodded and said enthusiastically, "Ok, great!" (Why did I say great?!) as my mind raced ahead to all the knee-bending in the sequence I had prepared.

Obviously, when you ask people about injuries you are supposed to follow-up with some helpful modifications, not just smile and say great. It's easier said than done, though. Even if you learned about it in teacher training, it is hard to recall the information on the spot, especially if you are a little nervous anyway. Other times, it will be something you have never heard of, something you have no information about at all, like that bruised coccyx.

This chapter is an introduction to common injuries and how to modify for them. I wanted to keep it short and simple so you can look up information in the moment you need it. For example, if someone tells you they have carpal tunnel five minutes before class starts, you can scamper off, flip to the carpal tunnel section, and scamper back with a few suggestions. Or just walk, scampering option.

Each entry includes the essentials of what to avoid and how to modify basic poses. If you are working with a special population or one-on-one with someone who has one of these conditions, you will want to research more. This short-and-sweet format, I hope, will help you cover your bases for some common issues that arise during your classes.

Arthritis

In general, yoga is good for arthritis, reducing pain and improving joint mobility. That said, go gentle at first and don't do anything that hurts. Arthritis varies among people, but in general, don't torque the joints in deep twists or extreme hip openers. Keep backbends mild, and keep the head in line with the rest of the spine. Avoid poses that require you to balance on one foot. Avoid bending the knees more than 90 degrees. Don't hold deep stretches for too long, as it can be difficult to get out of the pose.

Blood Pressure: High

Avoid inversions especially Headstand, Shoulderstand, and Plow because they increase the pressure to the head. In Legs Up the Wall, use a blanket under the head. Downdog is technically an inversion, so pay attention to how it affects you and take Child's Pose or Puppy Pose whenever needed. Beneficial poses for arthritis include seated forward folds, restorative poses, and gentle backbends like Supported Fish.

Blood Pressure: Low

Don't make sudden movements. Make sure you are breathing throughout practice, and inhale deeply whenever you are moving from down to up: lying to sitting, sitting to standing, upside down to right-side up. In particular, don't stand up too fast when transitioning from a Standing Forward Bend to Mountain Pose.

Hips: Replacement

Depends on the type of surgery: partial, total, posterior, anterior. Generally, don't go to extreme ranges of motion. If you practiced yoga before your surgery, don't force your body into poses that you used to be able to do if it hurts now. Roger Cole offers this advice from in *Yoga Journal* for practicing yoga after hip replacement.

Posterior: To avoid dislocation, avoid too much hip flexion, adduction, and internal rotation especially in combination, like Cow Face, Eagle, and Child's Pose. At the most conservative end, the recommendations are don't cross your legs for three to six months after surgery, and no flexion past 90 degrees for 12 months.

Anterior: Avoid abduction, external rotation, and hyperextension. For a year after surgery, avoid or be cautious with Warrior II, Triangle, Warrior I, Bound Angle, and Lotus. Keep backbends very mild, or skip them altogether.

Knee Pain

Use props. Pad the knees with a blanket, extra yoga mat, or special knee cushions you can find on-line. In Table, try a folded blanket under the shins so the kneecaps float an inch above the floor. Same for a low lunge. Back off a pose if you feel painful pulling in the sides or back of the knee. Find alternatives to full knee flexion (Puppy Pose instead of Child's Pose, Wide Leg Forward Bend instead of Bound Angle, Reclined Pigeon instead of Pigeon, Forward Fold instead of Squat). In Child's Pose, place a rolled up blanket or bolster between thighs and calves. Avoid hyperextending. In a knee-down lunge, move the back leg back so you're more on the top of the thigh than the kneecap. Don't straighten the leg all the way when there is pressure or weight on it. Keep a micro-bend in the knee in poses like Triangle and Half Moon Pose. Press hands into a block instead of your shin in Triangle.

Larger Bodies

Not that being larger bodied is a disability at all; it can just require modifications. Amber Karnes' two basic tips are: (1) widen and (2) move stuff out of the way. In folds, your feet can be as wide as your mat, and when going from standing to folding as in the Swan Dive, you can use your hands to tuck the flesh of your belly back toward your spine. In twists, take a more open version: don't worry about hooking your elbow in the "prayer twist" or crossing your foot as in Half-Lord-of Fishes. Also, as Karnes reminds, don't hesitate to simply move your breast or belly to the side in twists. In lunges, move the front foot wider and take blocks under the hands. Make space for the body in Vinyasa transitions. When moving from Down Dog to Forward Fold, walk hands back to feet instead of feet to hands, then walk to the top of the mat. When moving from Down Dog to a lunge, use blocks under the hands and step foot wider than hands.

Low Back Pain

Bend your knees when folding forward, when rising up to stand from a forward fold, and in Down Dog. Modify twists simply by not twisting as deeply. Reduce strain on the low back by gently stretching the hamstrings. Stretch the piriformis with Reclined Pigeon and the psoas with Supported Bridge. Strengthen the abdominals with Boat, Chair, and Plank. Use a bolster under the knees in *savasana*. Outside of yoga class, pay attention to how you move, sit, and stand. Take stretches throughout the workday.

Neck Injuries: Herniated Disc, Osteoarthritis, Severe Strains, Whiplash

Avoid extreme flexion, extension, and rotation in the cervical spine. Avoid inversions, especially Headstand. Instead of Shoulder Stand, do Supported Bridge Pose or pike the legs toward the ceiling with a block under the sacrum and a blanket under the head and neck. Keep the neck neutral to avoid hyperflexion in poses like Cobra, Camel, and Fish. In twists, stop at the thoracic spine, instead of turning the head to include the neck in the pose.

Pregnancy: First Trimester

Listen to your body, and take it easy if you are nauseous or fatigued. Avoid deep twists, which can interfere with placenta formation, and skip twists completely if you have miscarried in the past. Expand the pelvic region and create space for the baby with Reclining Hero, Bound Angle, and Reclining Big Toe Pose. Be careful not to overstretch, as the hormone relaxin is present from conception to after birth, and it makes all the connective tissues very flexible, so don't go as

deep as you can into poses, and avoid binds altogether. Avoid holding the breath for any length
of time in all stages of pregnancy.

Pregnancy: Second Trimester

Make space for your growing belly. In lunges,
take the front foot wider, bring your torso and
arms inside the leg, and use blocks under the
hands in lunges. Replace the traditional Plank to
chaturanga to Cobra sequence with Cat/Cow, or a
knees-down Plank and modified push up combination. Use blocks under the hands in Forward
Bend, and keep the feet wide. Bend the knees a
lot when rising up to stand from the pose. Avoid
lying flat on the belly: take a Table balance such a
Bird Dog instead of prone poses like Locust.
Avoid lying on the back without support for long
periods after 20 weeks. Avoid poses that isolate
the rectus abdominis muscles. Use *ujjayi* breath
to help support the back. Avoid twists that com-
press the abdomen. Continue to be careful not to
overstretch because of the hormone relaxin.
Avoid holding the breath for any length of time
in all stages of pregnancy.

Pregnancy: Third Trimester

Continue to be careful not to overstretch the lig-
aments, which are more flexible now in preparation for labor and delivery, especially the abdominals in side-bending poses and backbends.
Inversions are fine as long as they are well-sup-

ported, you can breathe well, and you are comfortable. Have a few go-to places to rest: Supported Child's Pose, Supported Hero's Pose, and Reclined Bound Angle Pose. Instead of *savasana* on your back, lie on your side, or on your back on a bolster with bent knees. Do Warrior II and Extended Side Angle to strengthen the muscles of the pelvis. Take Pigeon, Fire Log, and Bound Angle to stretch the hips. Asymmetrical forward folds can help position the baby's head down in the pelvis. Seated forward folds with wide legs and a concave back can be good to increase blood flow to the kidneys and lower body. Continue to avoid holding the breath for any length of time.

Pregnancy: Postpartum

Take it easy. Avoid core work stronger than Cow/ Cat for eight weeks after delivery. Progress to knee-down plank until three months postpartum, and the full plank after six months. At six to twelve months, progressively increase your core work on the ground and in poses like Boat.

Sciatica

Stretch the piriformis with Pigeon or Reclining Pigeon, Half Lord-of-the-Fishes-Pose, and Knees to Chest Pose. Strengthen the low back muscles with Locust Pose and Bridge Pose. Bend the knees in Standing Forward Bend, Downward Dog, and Seated Forward Bend.

Scoliosis

Scoliosis is complex and varies from person to person. A pose that helps one person might make things worse for you. Notice and respect the difference in abilities on the right and left sides. Unless you are working one-on-one with an instructor who has specialized training, listen to your body and avoid twisting too deeply toward the concave side of the spine, or stretching too much in the convex side.

Shoulder Injuries: Impingement, Rotator Cuff Injury, Old Dislocation

Modify any pose where the arms are lifted by keeping the hands in Prayer at the chest if the injury is recent or it hurts. Do Plank and Side Plank with knees down to help build strength without too much pressure on the shoulder. For Vinyasa, do a milder sequence of Inhale Downdog or Table > Exhale Cat to Child's Pose > Inhale Cow > Exhale Downdog or Table. Do Child's Pose if Downdog is too much.

Spine: Herniated Disc

Avoid rounding your spine. In seated poses, sit on the edge of a blanket or bolster to keep the spine long. Instead of seated forward bends, do Staff Pose which will strengthen core muscles and spinal posture. In Standing Forward Fold, either don't fold past 90 degrees without bending the knees, or avoid folding altogether. In Sun Salutation, do Chair Pose instead of Standing Forward Fold and Half Standing Forward Fold. Be very gentle in twists; don't go too deep.

Wrists: Carpal Tunnel Syndrome

Do not put pressure on the wrists. Skip Downdog and Plank. Instead, do these poses on the forearms or take Child's Pose. Avoid Vinyasa classes where it's more difficult to avoid weight-bearing on the wrists.

Wrists: Pain in Weight Bearing Poses

Spread your hands and distribute weight across the palms. Press into mound of index finger, mound of thumb, and the mound of the pinky. Use blocks under hands in Table, Plank, Downdog. If that doesn't help, go to the forearms in Downdog, Table, and Plank. Instead of "taking a Vinyasa," do Table > Cow > Cat > Downdog. Strengthen the core muscles so you can draw weight off the hands. Stretch the wrists in Table pose by turning the fingers to face your knees. Rest in Child's Pose when the wrists need a break. When there is persistent wrist pain, stick with stretching and strengthening for a week before returning to weight-bearing poses. Make a loose fist, palm up, and do curls with the wrist up toward the sky. Then turn the first so palm is down and do curls down toward the ground.

You Can Do it!

The longer you teach and the more students you encounter, the better you will be at helping people adjust and modify. You don't need to be an expert on everything right away. That's not realistic, and no one will think less of you for saying you need to do a little research and follow-up with an answer next time. In fact, those are key moments. This is a learning process. Every time a student tells you about an injury, make a note to research it when you get home. Also, talk to your students about their injuries. People are a valuable resource. You can learn a lot by asking students to describe how things feel, what helps, and what doesn't.

Finally, use your common sense when you don't know what to do. Help students avoid an extreme range of motion where there is pain in the body, provide props to cushion and support the body, and give reminders to stop if there is intense discomfort or sharp pain. Set a noncompetitive tone for your classes. Most importantly, remind your students to listen to their bodies because they are the real authority in their healing and recovery.

CHAPTER 9

Honest Marketing

"The best marketing doesn't feel like marketing."

- Tom Fishburne

Writing this book took me five years and many rounds of editing. One morning I sat down at the kitchen table to revise this particular chapter on marketing for yoga teachers, which had sat untouched on my Google Drive for three years. Three paragraphs in, I literally groaned and dropped my forehead on the table like a Cathy cartoon. "Are you okay?" Dan called from the other room.

I was not. The writing was bad—cliché and unimaginative. I sounded like a free webinar on "sales secrets." My advice on marketing was either obvious (hang flyers, make a website, social media) or jargon-y (hustle, target market, leads). Worse, the whole thing was infused with the philosophy of the marketing books I was reading at the time, which described marketing as a way to make yourself seem awesome and to play on people's fears and desires so they will give you money. For example, one book suggested, *Write a book! It doesn't matter what it's about or whether it's good. Just write one and then you can call yourself an author and people will see you as an expert!*

And that's why I wrote this book!

No, not really. Actually, I wrote it for the opposite reason. I wrote it because I felt like anything *but* an expert, and I believed that my genuine struggles could make other first-year yoga teachers feel less alone. I wrote it because I love to write. I wrote it because I believe that these are important topics for the future of yoga.

Maybe it's surprising, then, that these clever marketing people won me over with their tips and tricks—that there were whiffs of B.S. in the first couple of drafts of this marketing chapter. Or maybe it's not surprising. There is a lot of B.S. in our culture and we get used to the smell. It can be easy to buy into the philosophy of self-promotion for the sake of self-promotion, of success for the sake of success, going big for the sake of going big.

Still, reading the earlier version of this chapter at the kitchen table that morning, I saw traces of a more genuine marketing philosophy emerging, a more holistic approach focused on serving students rather than simply promoting yourself. In those pages, I saw the shimmer of a better, healthier philosophy on marketing that is much closer to my approach now, now that I have more experience teaching and more time to think about the right way to do it.

An hour later over breakfast, I explained all of this to Dan—how disappointed I was that the chapter was no good, how annoyed I was that I would have to rewrite the whole thing, how I felt embarrassed that I wrote it at all. "I think you can make that part of the chapter," Dan said, "the fact that a few years later your perspective on marketing has changed." Of course! Dan's so smart (he told me to put this in too). And so, here we are.

How I Was Wrong

After breakfast, I knuckled down and forced myself to read the whole cringy chapter, and I noticed three main things. The first was a problem to fix: the influence of bestselling self-help audiobooks that I was listening to at the time. Okay, fine, I still listen to self-help audiobooks! Okay, fine, I use most of my Audible credits on them! I am not ashamed; these books keep me motivated, focused, and inspired to dream about what is possible, but I have learned to take them with a grain of salt.

That's because authors in the genre tend to focus on getting what you want, achieving success, and making money without grounding the work in something substantial: a set of ethics, a moral code, a wisdom tradition. Of course, there are exceptions. *The Seven Habits of Highly Effective People* by Stephen Covey is the old school classic of the genre, and the whole message is to build your life on principles and character. In general, though, motivational books, or at least many of those that I have read, tend to focus on externally-validated success over service to something more satisfying.

The problem with approaching life as a game to win is that it feels hollow, and it's a poor basis for a marketing plan. Success for the sake of success inevitably disappoints. Self-promotion for the sake of self-promotion inevitably feels gross. I think that's why many of us in the yoga community resist marketing ourselves. It feels like a distraction. It feels ego-driven and out of alignment with the point of the whole thing.

In the years since I originally wrote this chapter, I have thought a lot about marketing, and have come to understand that marketing feels healthy when what you are selling is your service, not your image, when the message is about the real benefits of yoga for people, and not a glossy, unrealistic #yogalife dream. Understanding the distinction makes all the difference in the world.

When yogis do marketing by posting photos of themselves doing yoga, looking perfect, and gazing out into the middle distance, it gets dangerously close to how a cosmetics company markets make-up to consumers. *Buy this mascara and you will be beautiful, happy, effortlessly sexy.* While not overt, the subliminal message plays on our deepest insecurities, and the promise inevitably disappoints. The social media "yogalebrity" trend is unhealthy and unhelpful in the same way. Yoga isn't a quick fix for health and happiness; it's a process of learning to ride the waves of life's sadness and difficulty and pain with more grace and equanimity. But that's not very sexy.

So what's the alternative to image-based marketing? As I will explain in this chapter, you have another option. You can base your marketing efforts on what you are offering people through yoga. Talk about the actual benefits, and your classes specifically. This isn't hard when the product you are selling is yoga, because yoga works! It's so good for you! No, practicing yoga is not a quick fix, but does help you feel better. Inspire people to do something healthy and sustainable for themselves. Finally, concentrate on how you are serving others instead of promoting an image of yourself.

Back at the kitchen table, reading the earlier draft of this chapter, the second thing I noticed was my assumption that you have to strive for something large-scale—that marketing efforts were meant to propel you to the cover of *Yoga Journal* and to accumulate thousands of social media followers rather than simply lead healthy-sized, high-quality classes in your community. Back when I wrote it, I didn't have a lot of examples of successful yoga teachers who fall into the second category. I taught classes alone in rented studio space, away from home where I didn't have a community of peers as examples of how people make a living teaching yoga. Instead, I looked to YouTube yogis and famous teachers for career examples. With those as my main role models, I believed that success meant going big —lots of followers, teaching at *Yoga Journal* conferences, glossy Ayurvedic cookbook—which made marketing feel daunting and scary and out of my league.

Quick side note: if big is what you are aiming for—if you want to be a best-selling author or lead international sold-out retreats—you can figure out what you need to do to get there. If you have a burning desire to share something with the world, share it! As St. Thomas wrote, "If you bring forth what is within you, what you bring forth will save you. If you don't bring forth what is in you, what you don't bring forth will destroy you." Please, share your passion, share your gift, don't be afraid to use your voice!

Please understand that I am not encouraging you to stay small or keep quiet. The point I am trying to make is that marketing does not *have* to be something big if your dream is teaching three great classes a week at your local studio, while you continue to thrive at your regular job, spend time with people you love, and take one really good vacation every year with the extra income from teaching. In a few years, maybe you lead a retreat and some cool workshops. Instead of being glossy and big-scale, marketing can simply be a system for promoting, building, and sustaining those three classes. What I lay out in this chapter is an approach to help you do just that.

The third thing that I noticed when rereading the chapter is, thankfully, my ambivalence about the whole ego-driven, "go big" model of marketing. I wrote things like, "Many teachers, including me, don't like the idea of 'marketing yourself' and 'building your brand.' It feels...icky." But I would follow it with a resigned sentence like, "But it's just something you have to do if you want to succeed." It is this third thing upon which I built this more wholesome chapter on marketing. Yes, you do have to market yourself, but you do not have to do it in a way that feels icky. Here's how.

Marketing You Can Stand Behind

Here is my seven-step approach to marketing your yoga classes in a holistic, authentic, and sustainable way. Focus on service, on defining what you are *really* offering people, on connecting with your students, on cultivating a real community around your classes, and on building momentum that will last.

You don't need to take these steps in order; they can overlap. Also, expect things to shift and change as you grow and your career evolves: this is a continuous process and one you ultimately have to figure out for your particular situation. The purpose of this framework is to help you put your mind and heart in the right place to find real, lasting, satisfying success teaching yoga.

During the past few years, as my mindset has shifted toward service-based marketing, I discovered the business marketing coach George Kao and his "authentic marketing" approach. His videos and articles, at georgekao.com and YouTube, influenced my revision of this chapter. Kao offers a wholesome alternative to old-school manipulative marketing strategies to wear people down until you can sell them your thing. Instead, he says, focus on how your service can truly help people, and offer it from a place of open sincerity. His is a heart-centered approach that I think will resonate with many yoga teachers. I want to acknowledge George Kao for his influence on this chapter. Check him out.

Step 1: Know What You Are Offering

In order to have a clear and honest marketing message, you first must know what you are offering people. Of course, you are offering yoga classes, but I'm asking you to go deeper. What is the purpose of those yoga classes? What are you *really* offering? I am sure it's more than telling people how to do poses. When you know the answers to those questions, you can develop an authentic marketing message that you feel good about sharing.

If you don't yet have clarity on your purpose, revisit the mission statement questions from Chapter 2. Get out pen and paper, set the time for 30 minutes, and start writing. Try not to censor or edit yourself. Write in stream-of-consciousness. When the timer goes off, stop writing. A few days later, come back and do it again. Give yourself plenty of time to answer these: a couple of weeks or maybe even a couple of months. This is not light work. When you are ready, review what you wrote and tighten things up into a few sentences.

Once you understand your *why* and you have defined what you are *really* offering, your deeper purpose will come through in your marketing materials—naturally and effortlessly—whatever the medium. Whether you are sharing your message on your website, designing flyers, creating your business cards, posting on social media, or speaking with people face-to-face, your message will feel right when you are rooted in your purpose. Marketing won't feel icky when it comes from a place of truth, service, and passion.

Step 2: Don't Try to Get Everyone to Love You

I should get the title to this section tattooed on my knuckles. In the past, a big part of my motivation to teach great yoga classes was winning praise and admiration from others. It's still something I work to keep at bay. I can practically feel my brain light up when someone says sincerely after class, "That was great," or when my mom comes to my class and a regular student tells her, "Your daughter is an awesome teacher."

On the flip side, I feel awful when it seems like people aren't into the class or I am having an off day and not teaching my best. Over the past few years, I have gotten much better about letting those times roll off my back, but it can still be pretty rough. Sometimes when people walk out the door with a terse, "Thank you," I fight the instinct to shrink up and doubt myself, even if I thought the class was good. So as you read this, please know that I am writing it as much for myself as I am for you. We teach what we need to learn, after all.

If the first step of honest marketing is to know what you are offering and why, the second step is accepting that it won't resonate with every single person. Do that, and you free yourself to deliver something great for the people who *do* love it. Stand firm in what you are offering. Own it. Don't try to please every single person who unrolls their mat in your class. That's impossible.

It's impossible because yoga means different things to different people. Some people find peace and focus in a practice that is vigorous and fast-paced. Other people hate that; they don't even think it's "real" yoga. Many other people haven't thought about it much; they just want to move their bodies and breathe and feel better.

You will make yourself crazy trying to guess what everybody wants from your class. Worse, you won't succeed, and you will lose any clarity you have about what you are offering, and your marketing will be unclear and uncompelling.

A few years ago, I went to a jam-packed Saturday morning class at an Iyengar studio. The teacher was a regal older woman who had been teaching yoga for forty years, and my expectations for her class were high. That didn't last.

The teacher demanded precise alignment from the class, refusing to continue until every single person in the room followed her cues, and she pointed out specific students' mistakes to everyone else. In Cobra Pose, she directed, "Draw your outer heel toward your inner heel," which I suppose is a good cue, although a tricky one to execute. I guess not everyone followed the instruction, because she repeated louder, "Draw your outer heel toward your inner heel." A few seconds of silence. Then, "I'm not going to continue until everyone draws their outer heel in toward their inner heel!" *Jeeze!* I thought.

The class continued this way, and I hated it. I almost left but I didn't. When class ended, I was in a terrible mood and thinking a bunch of mean thoughts about the teacher and the studio. I thought about it the rest of the weekend, and eventually came to the conclusion there was nothing inherently wrong about the class. Well, we could get into a whole debate on whether most alignment rules serve people well, but we won't. The teacher clearly knew her stuff. She gave lots of information and modifications. She had a ton of experience. The studio was packed with people. It just wasn't my cup of tea.

You can't satisfy every student who comes to your class, even after 40 years of teaching experience. As a people-pleaser, that's hard for me to accept, but I'm improving. When I started out, I was desperate for every student to like my class. I would read one person's frown as a sign that the whole class sucked. I would add a dose of core work if a fit-looking woman came. When another yoga teacher came to my class, I would think, "Okay, what will impress her?" and I would teach the class based on what I thought she would like.

Now that I have more confidence as an instructor, I worry much less about everyone liking me. I don't take it personally if I'm not someone's cup of tea...most of the time. I understand that there are lots of different types of yoga and lots of different types of people...most of the time. To help brush it off my shoulders, I remind myself of an expression that one of my teachers uses, "I'm not for everybody, and neither are you." Amen.

Getting to this point in your teaching is an essential aspect of your personal and professional growth, and also an important part of marketing. You have to cultivate your individual style of teaching, clarify your philosophy behind it, find the people who resonate with it, and then focus on those folks. You have to do your best at what *you* do. In other words, be yourself! If you change for people who don't like you, you end up pleasing no one and losing the students who do like your classes. Be yourself, and your marketing message will be genuine and clear.

Step 3: Genuinely Care About Your Students

Originally, I called this section "Customer Service," but I changed the title because it didn't capture what I mean. "Customer service" makes me think of long rows of cubicles, full of people whose job it is to patronize unhappy callers. It makes me think of "the customer is always right," and that philosophy doesn't necessarily apply to our industry. The type of customer service I am talking about has an emphasis on the *service* part. Basically, Step 3 is an attitude of being kind and thoughtful, genuinely caring about your students, making people feel welcome and seen.

This is pretty simple. If you connect with your students as people, they are more likely to come back to your classes. Also, it feels good and it's the right thing to do. As you clarify your teaching style in Steps 1 and 2, you will start to attract regular students who resonate with you. When that happens, focus on serving them the best you can so they keep coming back. Giving people an exceptional experience in yoga class generates the most effective form of advertising: word of mouth. And, again, it feels good and it's the right thing to do.

Here are some ideas for delivering genuine customer service so you can build a great reputation for yourself and a strong student base for your classes.

Learn Students' Names

When you don't know someone's name, it's hard to connect with them. Someone recently told me, "If you're bad at remembering names, it's because you're not trying." It's true, remembering names is actually pretty simple. You just have to pay attention when they say it. It helps to repeat the person's name back to them, and come up with a way to remember the name, like "Shelly is so small she could live in a shell." It also helps to review your class roster and mentally repeat everyone's name during *savasana*.

Remember Things People Share With You

I talk to a lot of people every week and it can be hard to remember who I spoke with about what. A few weeks ago, I was talking to a regular student who was going on the weekend retreat led by another teacher at the studio. She was asking me about what she should bring, what the showers were like, how was the food. The next time I saw her, she said the retreat was great, and I blanked for a minute and said, "Oh, I didn't know you were going!" I could tell she was a little surprised that I didn't remember talking about it. It probably wasn't a big deal to her, but I felt badly, and it reminded me how important it is to really listen to people. Try to remember what students share with you about their vacations, their kids, their health issues, their jobs. This doesn't have to be deeply personal. You don't have to become their therapist—just friendly and thoughtful. You also don't have to force it. Let your student relationships grow naturally like you would with any other friendship.

Pay Attention to Students' Progress

As a new teacher, you can become absorbed with your own progress as a teacher and forget to look around the room at your students. If you have been teaching Half Moon Pose for a few weeks and you notice that a particular student has grown stronger and more balanced in the pose, tell her so. During class, you could just say, "Nice, Janet!" Or wait until after class to give her a high five and say good job. Same way, if a student tells you her wrists hurt in Downdog and you provide a few suggestions, ask if it helped the next time you see her. Encouraging words and thoughtful questions make a big difference.

Offer Something Extra

This isn't something you have to do every class, but it's nice to offer extra content once in a while. Make copies of handouts with a morning yoga routine. Give out little cards with inspirational quotes on them. Email a link to a video or an article. Recommend books. It shows that you care, and people like getting extra stuff.

Warmly Welcome New Students

It's pretty simple: when you have a new student make sure they feel welcome and have all the information they need. You may have been doing yoga so long that you don't remember what it's like to be a beginner. That was true for me until I visited a friend in Knoxville a few months ago, and she took me to her pole dancing class. I had never pole danced before (and I probably never will again), and I had no idea about the simplest things: where to put my shoes, which pole I should take, whether or not it was okay to talk before class started, where the bathroom was, who was the teacher. The experience reminded me to (1) be really friendly to new students who might be feeling intimidated and (2) explain logistics that might seem obvious to you.

Little Things Make a Difference

Make sure the room is clean and tidy. Don't get on your cell phone right after class. Smile at people. Make eye contact.

Step 4: Build Real Community

In his book *The Power of Habit*, Charles Duhigg tells a story about how the YMCA hired statisticians to analyze membership data and figure out what their members wanted from the gym. YMCA leaders assumed that their customers wanted top-line weight rooms and facilities, but that's not what the statisticians found. They were surprised to learn that while attractive facilities may have compelled people to join in the first place, it was not the main reason people continued to come. Instead, member retention was driven by emotional factors, such as whether employees knew members names or said hello when they walked in. Bottom line, people were more likely to keep coming if they felt a sense of community at the gym.

The YMCA study quantifies something that we intuitively know: people like to feel like they belong. If you create a feeling of belonging at your yoga classes, students will feel part of a group, and be more likely to keep coming back.

Step 4, Build Real Community, is a natural progression from Step 3, Genuinely Care about Your Students, and some of the ways you can enhance feelings of community overlap with the customer service tips from the previous section.

Ways to Build Community

- Again, remember students' names!
- Introduce students to each other and help them connect.
- Chat with your students before and after class.
- Tell your students about yoga-related community events.
- Consider starting a book club, a meditation group, or an "open gym" time.
- Socialize outside of class.

When I lived in Idaho, my yoga teacher was excellent at creating community at her studio. At my first class, Tasha introduced me to every other student by name. Over the weeks, we started going out for sushi or Thai after class once a week. On cold winter nights when I didn't feel like trekking seven blocks through the dark to the studio, I did anyway because I wanted to socialize. I also wanted to do yoga, of course, but I could have practiced at home. The community was irreplaceable.

I believe that one of the biggest benefits of modern yoga is a sense of belonging—discovering a place that is neither your work or home where people feel welcome, see familiar faces, receive inspiration, and make transformations.

At the studio where I work, there's a group of five of six retired people who always come to the midday classes at the studio. Over the past few years, I have watched them become a group of friends who go out dancing multiple times per week. Last night I overhead two other students—who are different ages, races and genders—discussing their plans to go skydiving together in the springtime. One of my best friends met her husband at the studio.

Yes, people do yoga to be fit and healthy. But don't underestimate the magnetic pull of real-life community in a world that is increasingly isolating. A sense of belonging is a huge factor in why people come back day after day; it brings a lot of joy and comfort to people. Personally, it is one of the things I love most about working at a studio. Cultivate community, and your classes will be robust and happy places to be.

Step 5: Focus on Teaching Your Best Classes

During my first few months of teaching, I worked like a maniac through lists of tasks, and spent all my free time making my website, designing flyers, and searching for more places to teach. It didn't leave much time to focus on actually planning the classes and learning more about yoga. As a result, the classes I taught were not as good as they could have been, and I didn't learn as much as I could have.

Certainly, marketing is necessary to grow your classes, get your name out there, and make a real go of it as a yoga instructor, but it shouldn't overshadow the actual teaching part. Focus on teaching the best classes you can, even if it's only for two people. I know some days it's easier to focus on your Facebook page or write website copy than it is to stay on your mat until you have planned a well-rounded class. But the time you spend developing your teaching skills is more important in the long run. People don't come back to your class because your flyer is attractive or because 50 people liked your post. They come back because you teach good classes and because they had a positive, inspiring experience

So if your class sizes are small right now, don't stress. Show up. Teach your best. Pour hard work, love, and clear intention into what you're doing and you're classes will be good. When your classes are good, people will keep coming, and they will tell their friends. Slowly and steadily, class attendance will climb and you will build a reputation as a good teacher. That is the cornerstone to building a healthy career.

Step 6: Create Your Marketing Materials

So far, I have included a lot about your mindset and attitude, and not much about specific ways to market your classes. There are a few reasons for that. First, you need to feel rooted in what you are offering and why you are offering it before you can create effective marketing campaigns. Second, how you approach marketing depends on your individual situation, your goals, your strengths, and your time. Last, I didn't want to make this chapter irrelevant by the time it's published by talking about a social media platform that no one uses anymore.

Instead, I will offer a handful of general ideas. These aren't wildly creative, but it's helpful to see on a page some basic options for getting started.

- Design a simple, functional website.
- Create a Facebook page, Instagram account, or YouTube channel specifically for your yoga classes and post consistently.
- Start building an email list and send out a monthly newsletter.
- Design flyers and business cards to post on bulletin boards.
- Record weekly videos to post online.

However you are approaching marketing, try to remain patient and grounded. Start slow and let things grow at their natural pace. You can't amass 1,000 Instagram followers in a year. Even if you could, would it be helpful? Stay clear on your deeper purpose, and craft all of your marketing efforts around it. When you do that, marketing is much less stressful.

Step 7: Risk Criticism

My friend recommended an online yoga workshop from a well-known teacher about sequencing, and when I looked it up on Facebook I did a double take of the photo. The teacher is lunging with one foot on a piece of driftwood, chest thrust forward and arms wide, dressed in an iridescent bra-top, many bracelets, and huge feather earrings. The description of the course was intriguing, if a bit opaque: "Learn to mirror the sequencing of the intelligent universe." I wasn't sure what that meant, and I did think she looked a little silly. Overall, though, my interest outweighed my skepticism, and I signed up.

But this is the internet, and there were plenty of people who saw the workshop and pounced. One man wrote, "Sequencing the intelligent universe? Lol. Please explain." Another person made fun of her outfit, and said it was cultural appropriation. Another guy simply posted the eye-roll emoji. Of course, along with the negative comments were lots of likes, shares, and people saying they were excited to take the workshop.

The cultural appropriation debate is one for another book. For now, my point is that when you put yourself out there, you will get negative feedback. Inevitably, people will disagree with you, misinterpret what you say, or project their own stuff onto what you are doing. You can't avoid it or control it. That's why it's essential to start your marketing process with a clear understanding about what you are offering and why, based on your values and your mission statement. That way, when people criticize or judge you, you can let it roll off your back, knowing that what you're doing is based on your values.

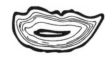

You Can Do it!

Marketing does not have to feel inauthentic or tacky. You can make it organic—a natural extension of your life and work, which grows at the same pace you do. When marketing is organic, you put less pressure on yourself and have more fun. But in order to do that, you need to have a clear understanding of your purpose. You need to stay rooted in your deeper why and avoid drifting into promotion for the sake of promotion. Make it about other people, not about you. With that foundation, you can make social media posts, flyers, short videos and newsletters that are effective, inspiring and useful for your audience. Amplify your message about what you truly want people to get from your classes. Focus on serving people instead of promoting yourself. It feels much better.

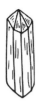

CHAPTER 10

Getting Down to Business

"So the question is not so much what are you passionate about. The question is what are you passionate enough about that you can enjoy the most disagreeable aspects of the work."

-Elizabeth Gilbert

The stereotype of yoga teachers is that we are a dreamy and naive bunch, especially when it comes to the topics of money, taxes, insurance, and the law. If this were *Friends*, we would be Phoebe.

I don't have to tell you that this stereotype is not accurate. Yoga teachers are professionals like anyone else. We are Chandler! In fact, yoga teachers often have to be *extra* organized, hardworking, and focused because you are often self-employed.

No one decides to be a yoga teacher because it's practical, or safe, or because it's what your parents always wanted. You choose it because it is your passion, which can sometimes mean that the business side of things takes a back seat. Not because you are living in outer space—there is just a lot to do.

This chapter establishes a foundation for the business of teaching yoga. It explains the basics of getting paid, paying taxes, buying insurance, and understanding liability. It is not an exhaustive explanation of the financial and legal aspects of teaching yoga, rather it is a starting point. Also, it is not legal advice! My brother-in-law who is a lawyer told me to make sure I included that. He also said to tell you to check your state and local regulations before making decisions about your money and your career. Ok, let's jump in.

Working as a Contractor vs. Employee

In the yoga world, teachers are often hired as independent contractors rather than employees. If you are hired to teach one class a week at a studio or a gym, you likely going to be classified as a contractor. But if you teach many classes at a studio and also work in management or the front desk, you might be hired as an employee.

The first major difference between contractors and employees is that you pay more in taxes as a contractor. I did not realize that when I was working as a technical writing contractor fresh out of college. When I got a letter from the IRS telling me I owed thousands of dollars, I panicked. I did not have the money, and I was used to getting money *back* from the government every year, not owing more. That year I learned the hard way that contractors are supposed to pay all the payroll taxes on their income, whereas employees split it with their employer. More on this later.

The second major difference is the level of control contractors are supposed to retain over how they do their jobs. Legally, contractors are supposed to have something that the IRS calls the Right to Control. On paper, it means that the studio owner shouldn't give you lots of specific instructions about how to do your job, or extra tasks in addition to just teaching the class. In reality, the Right to Control is fuzzy at most studios. It is common for studio owners to ask their contractors to do things in a specific way. It's not always a problem, but you need to be aware of it.

The third major difference is that employees enjoy some important legal protections that independent contractors do not, including unemployment insurance, workman's compensation, workplace anti-discrimination laws and the federally backed right to form a union, and overtime and minimum-wage laws.

It's an uncomfortable reality in the yoga world that often teachers pay the price of being a contractor, such as higher taxes, without reaping the benefits, such as more control over their work. In his book *Light on Law*, attorney and yoga teacher Gary Kassiah writes that many studios hire teachers as independent contractors to avoid payroll taxes, but treat them like employees anyway. Studios ask teachers to do a bunch of extra stuff like register new students, give studio tours, sweep and tidy up, and teach classes in a particular way. All this "create[s] strong presumptions that teachers are employees," says Kassiah, but they are still burdened with the higher taxes.

In the past, I have worked in this situation myself: paid as a contractor but treated as an employee. The studio owner, who I am very fond of, would email the teachers regularly with specific reminders about how to greet students, how to fold the blanket, whether or not to give adjustments, how the classes should be taught. I know that she just wanted to give students the best possible experience, and she was always really supportive and a great person to work for. I don't believe she was trying to take advantage of her workers, but the fact remains that she was treating her contractors very similar to employees, but not splitting the payroll taxes with us.

Still, I never talked to her about it—partly because it felt awkward, and partly because I only taught one class per week there and it didn't seem worth it. And if I am being honest, partly because I felt like yoga teachers aren't supposed to care about money.

Maybe after reading this chapter, you will make the same decision I did, and to leave things alone. Maybe you will make different decisions about where to work, how much money to ask for, or how much energy to invest in a particular opportunity. Maybe you will use it to have a conversation with your boss about your role at the studio and your job responsibilities. Whatever the case, you make better decisions when you have more knowledge, so let's get into it.

Contractors Withhold Their Own Taxes, Employees Do Not

When you are an employee, your employer withholds certain taxes from your paycheck. Most of us have worked as employees at some point, so you probably already know this. Imagine you are an employee at a yoga studio, and today is payday. You earned $500 during the pay period, but you receive a paycheck for less than that amount because your employer has already withheld taxes from it. Now imagine you are a contractor working for the same studio, and you earned the same amount—$500. In this case, the studio owner would write you a check for $500, straight up. She does not withhold any taxes; you have to do that yourself, and send the money to the IRS. Bottom line, when you receive a check for $500 as a contractor, you don't really have $500 to spend. Plan on withholding 25 to 30 percent of it for taxes to be safe.

Contractors Pay More in Taxes Than Employees

In addition to federal, state, and local taxes, we all pay taxes on the money we earn to fund Social Security and Medicare. This is called payroll tax. When you are an employee, you pay half and your employer pays half. When you are a contractor you pay the whole amount yourself. Earning $40 per class as an employee is not the same as earning $40 as a contractor because when you are a contractor you are paying double the amount of payroll taxes. Make sure you plan for that in your budget, and considering asking for a slightly higher pay rate if a studio wants to hire you as a contractor.

Contractors Pay Taxes Four Times a Year, Employees Pay Once

When you're a contractor, you send tax payments to the IRS four times a year instead of one time like employees. These payments are called quarterly estimated taxes, and you file them with the IRS in April, June, September, and January based on an estimation of how much money you will owe in taxes for the year. Most states require you to pay quarterly taxes as well. If you estimate too high, you will get a check for the amount you overpaid at the end of the year. If you estimate too low you might get a fine. You can determine how much you owe and how to make estimated tax payments on the IRS website in the Self-Employed Individuals Tax Center. In addition to the quarterly taxes, contractors file an annual return on April 15 like everyone else.

Contractors Can Take More Business-Related Deductions

In the winter of 2017, the Republican tax bill passed, and I had to scrap the section I had written on business deductions for independent contractors. It's still true that independent contractors can deduct more business-related expenses than employees, but the process and some rules are different.

The 2017 tax overhaul both simplifies and complicates deductions for the self-employed. It simplifies it because now sole proprietors deduct 20 percent of their revenue from their taxable income, instead of itemizing all their business expenses. It complicates it because there were a ton of changes for self-employed people and small business owners who take all their income from their business and file it on individual tax returns. The tax bill also affects how state and local taxes work for your business income and deductions. And of course, it's all subject to change if a new bill passes. So if you're working as a contractor, it's best to save all your receipts and work with a professional who can help you figure out your individual situation.

Contractors Retain the Right to Control

As I said earlier, clients (i.e. the studios) are not supposed to tell independent contractors how to do their job in much detail. If they do, the worker should be classified as an employee, not a contractor. The IRS uses a 20-factor Right to Control Test to determine whether a person is functionally an employee or a contractor. The test looks at things like whether the business owner provides training for the worker, whether the worker uses equipment provided by the owner, whether the owner sets the worker's schedule, and whether the worker depends on the owner for most of their income. Answering yes to any of those questions nudges the definition closer to "employee," but a single "yes" doesn't automatically make the worker an employee. Rather, the IRS looks at the big picture, the answers to all the questions together. Not that the IRS is going to come in and tell your boss to hire you as an employee—they don't have time for that. Rather, it's up to you to talk to the studio owner about it if the answer is "yes" to most of these questions.

How to Use This Information

One reason that studios hire teachers as independent contractors even though they are functionally employees is that it's cheaper. Studio owners don't have tax obligations on contractors. It's a pervasive issue not only in the yoga industry but in the wider workforce. Many big companies now hire janitors as contractors, instead of employees, which sucks for the janitor, who not only pays more in taxes but also lacks employment benefits like workman's compensation, health insurance, and the right to unionize.

It's difficult to know how to navigate it. As a yoga teacher, especially a brand-new one, you don't have much leverage. If you assert your Right to Control to a studio owner by refusing to sweep or teach class according to their instructions, or if you tell them you'll only take the job if you are classified as an employee, the studio owner may just find another person to hire.

Still, knowing the distinction between a contractor and employee may help you make better decisions about where and how to work. You may decide you only want to work for studios that hire employees for the ease, simplicity, and stability. You may choose to run classes independently, where you can teach classes exactly how you want to. You may try to negotiate a higher pay rate when a studio owner designates you as a contractor while making employee-style requirements. You're not a bad yogi for being smart, being strategic, asking for more money, or asserting your rights.

Choosing a Business Entity

If you are a contractor, here are three ways you can do it, and a brief summary of the advantages and disadvantages of each. Check the specific regulations where you live.

Sole Proprietorship

A sole proprietorship is a business that legally has no separate existence from its owner. Income and losses are taxed on the individual's personal income tax return. Contractors are automatically a sole proprietors.

Advantage: It is simple—usually you don't need to register with the government, pay any fees, or file paperwork. You pay taxes on your individual Schedule C and a 1040 Form.

Disadvantage: Your personal assets are tied to your business. If your business is sued and the plaintiff wins, you are personally responsible for paying the settlement. Likewise, if your business fails, you personally would declare bankruptcy.

Employees vs. Independent Contractors

Question	Employee	Contractor
Which IRS tax form is used?	W-2	1099, if more than $600 earned
Are certain taxes withheld from paycheck?	Yes	No
Who pays taxes on the worker's income?	Employer pays matching share of Medicare and Social Security tax.	Worker pays all state and federal taxes on income.
When does the worker file taxes?	Once per year by April 15.	Quarterly in April, June, September, January.
Can the worker deduct business expenses?	No	Yes
Eligible for benefits?	Depends	Not usually
Are you covered by labor laws?	Yes	Not all
Does the employer retain Right to Control?	Yes	No

DBA (Doing Business as)

Operating under a DBA is the same as a sole proprietorship except you do business under a fictitious name like "Yoga by Becky," which you register with the government.

Advantage: You create a brand name without having to create a company or an LLC.

Disadvantage: It's a bit more work; you need to register a DBA name with your county clerk or your state government. Procedures vary by state, and a few states actually don't actually require you to register your DBA, so check the regulations where you live.

Limited Liability Corporations (LLCs)

Unlike a sole proprietorship or a DBA, an LLC is a separate legal entity from the person or people who own it. The procedures for forming an LLC vary by state.

Advantage: You legally separate your personal assets from your business assets. If your LLC goes into debt or gets sued, you are not personally liable. For example, if you get a loan to open a yoga studio, and you default, the bank usually cannot seize your home or your personal assets to satisfy the debt. It can only seize business assets like money in your business accounts and business equipment. Likewise, if you need to declare bankruptcy, the business declares bankruptcy—not you personally.

Disadvantage: Forming an LLC is more expensive and time-consuming than a sole proprietorship. Depending on where you live, you will pay annual fees, and you will also need licenses and permits. You have to comply with various state regulations, including rules on naming your LLC and filing an Article of Incorporation document with your Secretary of State. Also, it's not a magic shield from all liability. Actually, some creditors might require you to personally guarantee your LLC's loans and credit cards anyway, and an LLC won't protect you against negligence lawsuits or if you do something intentionally fraudulent, illegal or reckless. So you can't create an LLC and then rest easy thinking you'll never be liable for anything ever.

Liability 101

Students who get injured in a yoga class sometimes sue the teacher or the studio for negligence, and although it's never happened to someone I know, it can happen. Rates of injuries in yoga classes are on the rise, or at least they are getting reported and recorded more frequently, so it's smart to protect yourself in case a student gets hurt in your class and decides to sue you. Liability waivers and personal liability insurance are the two main ways to do that.

Make a Liability Waiver

If you are running your own classes, you will need to have a liability waiver. To understand liability waivers, you first need to know the distinction between gross and ordinary negligence.

Gross negligence is when someone is aware of a problem and fails to correct it. If a student tells you there is broken glass on the studio floor and you don't clean it up, and later a woman cuts her foot, you might be found liable for gross negligence. You were aware of the problem, you had a responsibility to fix it, and you did not fix it.

Ordinary negligence is "a failure to act as a reasonable person according to the standards of care of your profession." For example, if someone tells you they have a herniated disc and you offer no information or modifications, and the person further damages their spine during practice, you *could*—maybe—be sued for ordinary negligence.

An attorney reading this might stop me right here and point out that negligence is complicated and nuanced, and varies case-by-case. Well, get out of here, ya fancy-schmancy law-yer! We are going for broad strokes here.

The point is that most liability waivers, even the best ones, apply only to ordinary negligence and not gross negligence. You can't write a waiver that includes the "reckless and intentional acts" that constitute gross negligence because most states say that liability for "reckless and intentional acts" can never be waived. In the example of the glass on the floor, a waiver would not protect you in court if the student decided to sue you. I repeat, liability waivers only apply to ordinary negligence.

If you work for a studio or a gym, they likely already have a student liability waiver, but if you run classes on your own, you will need to make one. There are plenty of good templates online that you can use, just make sure it's specific. If a person doesn't understand what he or she is actually waiving, the waiver will not hold up in court. A strong waiver includes:

- A description of the activity.
- That the signer has a full understanding of the nature of the document.
- That the signer knows the specific risks.
- That the signer has voluntarily chosen to assume the risks.
- That the signer agrees not the hold the institution liable for consequences of his or her participation in the described activity.

Of course, you can get a lot more specific with evaluating your liability wavier, and if you are planning on opening your own studio or running your own classes you probably should get legal help with it.

There is a 2008 article "Evaluating Your Liability Wavier," on the website Athletic Business that includes the criteria for a 100-point test to measure the strength of liability waivers. But liability laws differ from state-to-state, so if you have questions you should check your local laws and ask a professional attorney. This information is not intended as legal advice, rather as helpful information from another yoga teacher. Use it as a foundation, not the complete picture.

Buy Liability Insurance

You probably are aware that yoga teachers can—and often must as a condition of being hired somewhere—purchase personal liability insurance. If you get sued by a student who gets hurt in your class, the insurance company would (hopefully) contribute to the court costs and settlements. Like registering with Yoga Alliance, being insured is not a *legal* requirement for teaching yoga, but studios and gyms where you work might require you to have it.

Even if it's not required, it's a good idea to buy a policy. They are not expensive, and even though the probability of a lawsuit is low, it does sometimes happen.

In 2013 Alec Baldwin's wife Hilaria Thomas was involved in a civil suit after a student lost his balance in a headstand and crashed into a plate-glass window in her sixth-floor studio in Manhattan. Thankfully, he didn't fall to the East 12th Street sidewalk below, but he did cut his leg badly on the shattered glass. In the suit, the student claimed Hilaria put students in "extreme danger" because her class was too full—with the mats only an inch or two apart—to safely do headstands near the glass windows.

I looked it up, and the plaintiff actually sued the owner of the building where the studio was located—not Hilaria Thomas or the studio Yoga Vida. The distinction between these three separate entities—the building owner, the studio and the teacher—brings us to an important point about liability insurance at studios and gyms.

Most studios and gyms do have their own insurance policies, so you might assume that if you work for one, you are protected under their umbrella, but that's not always true. In fact, yoga studios typically require teachers to have their own liability insurance. If you work somewhere as an employee, the insurance policy might cover your employer but only provide minimal protection for you personally. And if you teach classes somewhere as an independent contractor, it's safe to assume that the studio policy will not cover you.

Like I said, having liability insurance is a good idea, and many employers want you to have it, but it's not required by law. I used to teach in a donation-based yoga collective run by a badass lady who split her time teaching yoga and working on an organic farm, and she didn't have insurance. The whole operation was frugal in a way that I loved but may not have been legally sound. To save paper, she made a single copy of the liability waiver for people to sign instead of making a separate copy for each student. As a sign-in sheet, we used a mini spiral notebook that looked like a freebie from a college orientation in 2004. She taught a few classes a week, mostly to students that she knew, and she told me that she would rather take what she perceives to be a very small risk than spend the money. I am not recommending that you teach yoga without liability insurance, only letting you know that it's an option for you bad boys.

As far as specific policies, there are several comparable options for yoga teacher liability insurance. The cost and coverage are often based on how many hours a week you teach. Some like Yoga Alliance and *Yoga Journal* come bundled with memberships. Shop around and compare policies from Yoga Alliance, Yoga Journal, the National Association of Complementary and Alternative Medicines (NACAMS), beYogi, Hiscox, and more.

Register with Yoga Alliance

If you graduated from a Yoga Alliance accredited teacher training, you can register with Yoga Alliance. It's a good first step to take after you finish teacher training, so naturally, I put it at the end of the book!

If you are ready to start teaching, but you aren't sure what your next step should be, you could get the ball rolling by registering with YA.

If you choose to register with Yoga Alliance, you will be listed in the public directory, you can put RYT (registered yoga teacher) credentials behind your name, and stick the little YA logo on your business card. You also get a discount at some retailers and access to a research database and video lectures.

I want to note, though, that you are not legally *required* to register with Yoga Alliance to teach professionally, at least not as of the time of publication. The registration fee isn't cheap at $100 initially and $55 annually. Membership can lend credibility if you're looking for jobs, but unlike a lawyer's bar association, it is not an industry standard. Studio owners or gym managers may prefer it, but others may not check, or notice, or care. So if you don't have an extra $100 to spend, if the benefits aren't worth the dues for you, or if you are skeptical of the whole thing, you can decide not to register.

If you do register, you must report at least 45 teaching hours and 30 hours of continuing education after three years. You can learn how to log hours and what qualifies as "continuing education" on the Yoga Alliance website. This is not an immediate concern for new teachers, but you can avoid scrambling three years from now if you keep track of hours starting now.

Keep Good Records

Speaking of tracking your teaching hours—keep good records. This is especially important if you are running the classes independently, charging money, and paying rent, but it's also wise if you work at a studio, gym, or as a volunteer. Keep a spreadsheet listing each class you teach. Include the date, time, location, style of class, and any additional notes you want to make. You could also choose to include how much money you made, or something in particular you learned from the experience.

It may seem tedious, but it's good to know how many classes you have taught in your career. You can include the information on resumes and your Yoga Alliance profile. Plus, it's gratifying to see your experience accumulate. The day I realized I had taught over 1,000 Vinyasa classes, I felt pretty cool. Then when I taught a workshop on how to teach all-levels Vinyasa, I could say, "I have taught more than 1,000 Vinyasa classes, guys!" and everyone thought I was very cool.

It's also a good idea to keep track of all your continuing education, including workshops, on-line courses, retreats you attend, and weekend-long training. This type of stuff adds up too and makes it easier to write a robust resume.

You Can Do It!

You know this by now, right? You got this.

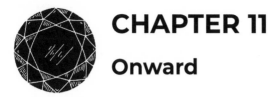

CHAPTER 11
Onward

"Those of us who are writers work out our stuff in public, even under the guise of pretending to write about someone else. In other words, we try to teach what it is that we really need to learn."

-David Brooks

This might be the only yoga book in history to wrap up with a quote from conservative commentator David Brooks, but it's how I feel about this project.

When I finished the first draft of this book and started quietly telling people about it, my spiel was that I wanted to publish it to help other new yoga teachers, like the whole thing was one big selfless act of service.

From the bottom of my heart, I hope this book helps you, but if I am being honest, I wrote this book for me. Of course I did. I wouldn't have spent hundreds of hours, gotten out of bed at 5 am, obsessed over the thing, made my shoulders tense and my eyes sore if I wasn't getting something out of it. I wouldn't do all that for you; I don't even know you! Just kidding, I love you. Writing about my story, my mistakes, my lessons, my progress, and my insecurities was how I got through a difficult period of being a new teacher, having no idea what I was doing.

Isn't that how we learn from each other though? One person gets honest and vulnerable about their experience, they talk about it, and it is helpful for others. It's helpful because it makes you feel less alone when things are hard. It's helpful because you can learn from their mistakes. It's helpful because sometimes the other person is able to distill into words the thing that has been germinating inside your mind but hasn't quite come to the surface.

Plus, I love making things, and then proudly showing those things to my parents.

In the end, I do hope that reading this book will help you. Of course I do. Now that I have finished it, I am thinking not of myself but of you —you who are reading this right now, who so badly wants to bring forth what's inside you, share your practice with others, teach amazing yoga classes, make the world a little better, but who is also freaking out a little. You feel so ready, but you don't know where to start. You feel like you were born to do this, and at the same time, you feel like a total fraud. It's a crazy place to be, I know, and if nothing else, I hope this book gives you company there and shows you the path out.

Resources

Next Steps: A Checklist for
New Yoga Teachers

After you graduate teacher training, it's actually not that important what you do first. The important thing is that you do *something*: it's good for your momentum and it's good for your confidence. Here are ten ideas for getting off your butt and getting started. You definitely don't have to do these things in order.

- Register with Yoga Alliance, if you want
- Write a short bio (see page 170)
- Draft your mission statement (see page 169)
- Create a simple resume (see page 170)
- Let people know via email or social media that you are a yoga teacher now
- Brainstorm ten places you could teach classes, volunteer, or paid.
- Contact or visit each place you've identified.
- Buy liability insurance
- Find a class with an experienced teacher you can attend every week
- Spend 30 minutes journaling on your long-term goals and dreams

Prompts for Drafting Your Mission Statement

- What's the point of yoga?
- What are your core values?
- How do you hope people feel after class?
- Why are you a yoga teacher?
- What is the role of a yoga teacher?
- Which aspects of yoga are you most excited to share?
- In teaching, what does your best effort look like?
- What are your best qualities as a human?
- Describe a great yoga class in three words.
- What do you hope people say about your classes?

Prompts for Plotting Your Destination

- Do you want teaching yoga to be your only job, a part-time job, or an "honored hobby?"
- What type of classes (big groups, small groups, privates) do you enjoy teaching the most?
- How many classes per week do you want to teach?
- Do you want to work for yourself, like an independent contractor at many different places, or as part of a team, employed at one studio?
- How much income do you need to support the life you want?

- Identify any special interests, such as prenatal yoga, yoga for trauma, yoga for youth, restorative yoga, yoga in the workplace.
- Write out a day-in-the-life of your dream job. Be as specific as possible.

Prompts for Writing Your Bio

- Where did you complete your 200-hour training?
- What styles of yoga do you teach?
- What's your yoga story? When and how did you start practicing? Keep this brief.
- What do you hope your students get out of your class? How do you hope they feel afterward?
- Do you have any other specialized training or experience that relates to yoga?
- Say a little something about your personal life, like what you like to do in your free time?
- How can people contact you?

What To Include on Your Resumé

- An objective—a simple and clear statement on why you want to teach yoga at that studio
- A profile—similar to your bio, describe your teaching philosophy and style
- Your teacher training—list your 200-hour program, its philosophy, and key learnings
- Additional trainings—workshops, online courses, meditation classes, etc.
- Work experience teaching yoga—any classes you have taught, paid or unpaid
- Other relevant work experience

Post-Class Reflection Template

Date _ _ _ _ _ _ _

Class _ _ _ _ _ _ _ _ _ _ _

Which two teaching skills I am focusing on right now? How did I consciously try to improve on them today?
1.

2.

What are three things that went well in that class?
1.

2.

3.

What could I improve next time?

Any other lessons learned or things to remember?

Sample Interview Questions

- Tell me about your 200-hour training.
- What did you like most about your training? What do you think your 200-hour training lacked?
- Describe your teaching style.
- Describe your yoga practice.
- How would you modify an intermediate or advanced level class for a beginner student?
- Tell me about a time when you had to give special modifications or accommodations to a student.
- What type of classes are you most comfortable teaching?
- How did you hear about the studio?
- Why do you want to work here?
- What type of support do you want from us, as a studio?

Recommended Reading

Not necessarily all yoga titles, these are books that have inspired me during the past few years.

Adele, Deborah. *The Yamas and the Niyamas: Exploring Yoga's Ethical Practice.* Duluth, Minnesota: On-Word Bound Books, LLC, 2009.

> You may have read this book as part of your teacher training. It's a pretty popular book and for good reason. I love this book; I recommend reading it again and again. Deborah Adele writes about the "ten jewels" of yoga in a way that makes you want to live an impeccable life. Read it for yourself to stay in a wholesome state of being, and read short passages to your students in class.   Start a book club with it. Teach a workshop around it. Keep it on your nightstand.

Brooks, David. *The Second Mountain: The Quest for a Moral Life.* Random House, 2019.

> David Brooks is a conservative columnist and pundit, and he published this book in 2019 after a rough few years during which his marriage fell apart, his political party became unrecognizable to him, and his kids went to college. He did still have a very successful career but felt empty. The first mountain is what society tells us to

climb: traditional monetary success, developing a good reputation, and rising to prominence in our field. But then we realize it's not actually fulfilling. The second mountain is what actually brings us joy: service to others, giving of ourselves, commitment to something greater than ourselves. I recommend it because I think it is easy as yoga teachers to get sucked into the Instagram life, competing for the biggest classes, and basing success on how what other people say about you. This book is a great reminder to come back to your heart, and to come back to service.

Brown, Brené. *Daring Greatly: How the Courage to Be Vulnerable Transforms the Way We Live, Love, Parent, and Lead.* Penguin Random House, 2012.

Brené! Brené Brown started her career as a shame researcher at a university, and more recently she has brought what she has learned about "wholehearted living" to a wider audience. Combining research and storytelling, Brené explains how you can work through your mental barriers to doing your life's work. It's a book about being brave, and overcoming your fear of failure, criticism and not being good enough. It will inspire you to move forward with courage, even if you are scared and you don't feel ready.

Clark, Bernie. *Your Body, Your Yoga: Learn Alignment Cues That Are Skillful, Safe, and Best Suited To You.* Wild Strawberry Productions, 2016.

> This one is more of a reference book than a sit-down-and-read book after you get past for the first few chapters. Clark explains how much variation there is in the human body, and why we as yoga teachers might want to forget a lot of what we learned in teacher training. Alongside his teacher Paul Grilley, Bernie Clark is an advocate for using functional rather than aesthetic alignment principles. In other words, don't focus on how the pose looks, focus on how it feels. Don't worry about getting all of your students into some standard textbook version of the pose, describe to them what is the target and let them feel it out in their own bodies. It will change how you teach and think about yoga forever.

Cope, Stephen. *The Wisdom of Yoga: A Seeker's Guide to Extraordinary Living.* Bantam, 2007.

> I relied heavily on this book when I taught a workshop on living yoga "off the mat," and Stephen Cope is the reason I decided to do my 300-hour training at Kripalu. This book is easy to understand because he uses characters and stories to explain philosophy that can otherwise be esoteric and difficult to apply to modern life. For yoga teachers, it is a great tool to help you

figure out how to weave philosophy into your class themes in a way that is relatable and understandable.

Fields, Jay. *Teaching People, Not Poses: 12 Principles for Teaching Yoga with Integrity.* CreateSpace Independent Publishing Platform, 2012.

> I lent my copy of this great little book to a friend, and I think she lost it during a move. I will buy another copy of it on Amazon, though, because it is sweet and sincere and comforting. Jay Fields reminds readers what's really important: being yourself, connecting with students, teaching from your own experience. A book to reread whenever you need a pick-me-up.

Gilbert, Elizabeth. *Big Magic: Creative Living Beyond Fear.* Riverhead Books, 2015.

> More than most people, Elizabeth Gilbert, the author of *Eat, Pray, Love,* knows what it's like to put yourself out there, the good and the bad. After *Eat, Pray, Love* was published, many people wrote to her saying that it had literally saved their lives. But lots of other people ridiculed her, saying her book was the worst thing ever. In some ways, *Big Magic* is her response to that crazy time in her life. It will encourage you to express your creativity and your passion and to not let the fear of criticism hold you back.

Little, Tias. *The Yoga of the Subtle Body: A Guide to the Physical and Energetic Anatomy of Yoga.* Shambala, 2016.

Take this puppy one chapter at a time. It's potent. Tias Little explains better than almost anyone the bridge between the physical body and the psycho-spiritual body. I have gleaned tons of beautiful verbal cues from this book. Tias Little phrases things in the most poetic and imaginative way. Because each chapter is focused on an area of the body or a chakra, I have found it useful to make my theme for the week "rooting," for example. Then I reread the chapter on the feet incorporate his ideas and descriptions into my class plan.

Pink, Shel. *Slow Beauty: Rituals and Recipes to Nourish the Body and Feed the Soul.* Running Press, 2017.

This might seem like a random pick, which fits because I randomly picked it from the library shelves one summer afternoon. It's a manifesto of taking pleasure in life, slowing down, incorporating rituals into daily life, and understanding that beauty comes from the inside out. With meditation practice, movement ideas, recipes for nourishing food, and DIY beauty products, it's just right for us crunchy yoga teachers who need some self-care.

Acknowledgments

Deepest love and thanks to my husband, Dan. Thank you for coming to all those early yoga classes to help me be less nervous. Thank you for affirming me with sincerity each and every time I need it. Thank you for reading so many drafts of this book with care, attention, and interest. Thank you for knowing all the grammar rules and all about writing good. Thank you for making me laugh so hard every day. Thank you for loving me so well. The life we are building together is one that makes me content and proud.

Infinite gratitude to my parents, Kevin and Trish. Thank you for teaching me the importance of hard work, practice, showing up, and believing in myself. Thank you for always telling me that I can learn to do anything in the world as long as I can read the directions, and for creating for me a childhood of exploration, discovery, and fun wrapped in a cocoon of safety and love. Thank you for always being excited to see what I make. Thank you for all the sacrifices you made to create the conditions for me to thrive. I love you very much.

Many heartfelt thanks to the friends who gave me thoughtful feedback, read drafts, cheered me on, and pushed me to keep going when I wanted to quit. Thank you to Lindsay Wolff: my bosom buddy and inspiration machine. Thank you to Brenna McDermott: a friend for life and editor extraordinaire. Thank you to Ashley Sturm: my coach and sunshine during the final stretch. Thank you to Alana Gaspard: a kind and beautiful person who told me that she needed to hear the message in this book at a time when I had abandoned it. Thank you Stacy Broussard for giving me feedback on tricky chapters. Thank you to my Soul Goals sisters: Lizzie Salsich, Erin Gruenburg, Melanie Hessler, and Katie Adelia who listened, affirmed, and helped me believe in this idea.

Thank you to my yoga family at Urban Breath Yoga in St. Louis. Thank you, Cathleen Williams, for making my dream job possible and supporting my continuing education. Thank you to all my co-workers who make me excited to come to work and inspire me to be the best teacher I can be. I love being on a team with you. Thank you to my community of yoga students! I am so grateful for you. When I have had a bad day, you lift me up.

Thank you to all my teachers, especially the world-class staff at Kripalu Center for Yoga and Health. Thanks to all my teachers over the years, whether we are friends or have never met, whether you teach me in person or through your books and videos. Thank you for your dedication, wisdom, and passion for a practice that heals and transforms.